Liposomes - Recent Advances, New Perspectives and Applications

Edited by Rajeev K. Tyagi

Published in London, United Kingdom

Liposomes - Recent Advances, New Perspectives and Applications
http://dx.doi.org/10.5772/intechopen.102167
Edited by Rajeev K. Tyagi

Assistant to the Editor: Nikunj Tandel

Contributors
Ujjawal Sharma, Bunty Sharma, Sampan Attri, Jyoti Syal, Iman M. Alfagih, Michał Chudy, Paweł Krysiński, Edyta Maroń, Munitta Muthana, Alessandra Iscaro, Faith H.N. Howard, Zidi Yang, Fern Jenkins, Dumitru Popescu, Alin Gabriel Popescu, Abdul Hafeez, Shazia Afzal Usmani, Rajeev K. Tyagi, Prakriti Sharma, Mili Mehta, Nikunj U Tandel

First published in London, United Kingdom, 2023 by IntechOpen
IntechOpen is the global imprint of INTECHOPEN LIMITED, registered in England and Wales, registration number: 11086078, 5 Princes Gate Court, London, SW7 2QJ, United Kingdom

British Library Cataloguing-in-Publication Data
A catalogue record for this book is available from the British Library

Additional hard and PDF copies can be obtained from orders@intechopen.com

Liposomes - Recent Advances, New Perspectives and Applications
Edited by Rajeev K. Tyagi
p. cm.
Print ISBN 978-1-80356-365-7
Online ISBN 978-1-80356-366-4
eBook (PDF) ISBN 978-1-80356-367-1

Meet the editor

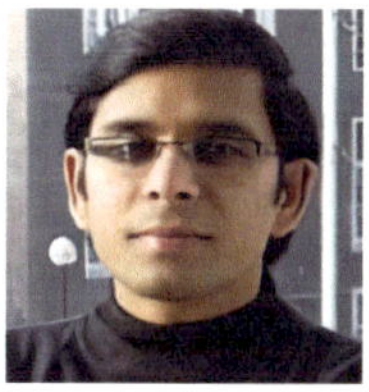

Dr. Rajeev K. Tyagi has been leading a group at CSIR-Institute of Microbial Technology, Chandigarh, India. He obtained his Ph.D. in 2011 at the Biomedical Parasitology Unit, Institute Pasteur, Paris, where he developed a long-lasting, stable and straightforward laboratory animal model (humanized mouse model). Dr. Tyagi's post-doctoral work was carried out at the University of South Florida, Augusta University and Vanderbilt University Medical Center (VUMC), USA, where he used the humanized mouse model as a tool to study the infectious disease *P. falciparum* and inflammatory diseases (*P. gingivalis,* colitis). His current research group is working on the development of human-liver chimeric mice for huHep transplantation, the antimalarial and anti-inflammatory potential of oleuropein has been explored in the asexual blood stage infection of *P. falciparum* and in-vitro models of inflammation (LPS-stimulated human THP-1 macrophages), and. on formulation and characterization of nanoscale drug carriers to deliver methotrexate (MTX) and aceclofenac in the treatment of rheumatoid arthritis, breast cancer and other inflammatory diseases.

Contents

Preface

As teachers of immunobiology, we have become increasingly aware of the lack of detailed material in many undergraduate medical courses on experimental approaches to drugs and their effective delivery in the treatment of cancers and infectious diseases. This book provides much-needed information about lipidic nanoscale carriers to deliver drugs to treat cancers and infectious diseases, their mechanism of action, and the pressing issue of evolving drug resistance.

The book addresses the perceived needs of both medical school and undergraduate curricula by synthesizing key concepts in the rapidly advancing and dynamic field of drug delivery. The choice of what is most important is based on what is most clearly established by experimentation, what our students find puzzling, and what explains the efficiency of drugs to treat cancers, infectious and inflammatory disorders. In-vitro and animal models are used to study the mechanism of action of existing and novel drugs. Lipid-based nanoparticles and their engineered versions are used for the effective delivery of drugs and candidate antigens. These drug carriers are of the utmost importance in reducing cytotoxicity while maintaining maximum therapeutic effects and the antigenic potential of drugs and antigens. This book discusses the role of nanoscale drug carriers in the delivery of antigens and vaccine candidates for the maximum therapeutic effect and vaccination potential against infectious diseases as well as cancers. It is a timely addition to the existing literature on delivery vehicles and a useful resource for those working in the field of the immunobiology of cancers and infectious diseases.

Rajeev K. Tyagi
Division of Cell Biology and Immunology,
Biomedical Parasitology and Nano-immunology Lab,
CSIR-Institute of Microbial Technology (IMTECH),
Chandigarh, India

Section 1

Liposomes as a Drug Carrier

Chapter 1

Introductory Chapter: Liposome - A Versatile Tool for Drug Delivery in Nanobiomedicine

Prakriti Sharma, Mili Mehta, Nikunj Tandel and Rajeev K. Tyagi

1. Introduction

Liposomes are lipid mono- and bilayered structures made up of cholesterol and phospholipid and entrap lipophilic or hydrophilic agents. The lipophilic agents have higher affinity towards phospholipid bilayer allowing their encapsulation within the lipid bilayer whereas the hydrophilic compounds are entrapped in the liposome central cavity [1]. Although size of liposomes ranges from nm to μm, widely used liposomes for various biomedical applications are in the range of 50 to 450 nm. Further, numerous experimental evidences confirm the role of liposomes as an emerging carrier for an effective drug delivery due to their resemblance with the cell that in turn allowed incorporation of range of drugs [2, 3].

These nanoscale drug carriers are demonstrated to be advantageous for promoting the biodistribution of drugs to target site-specific sites in the experimental animals, stabilizing therapeutic drugs, and overcome the physiological barriers. This ultimately allows these carriers to distribute the encapsulated substances to target areas efficiently and limit the systemic toxicity. The clinical translation of liposome-assisted drug delivery systems has advanced gradually over the past 5 decades, and generated wealth of information useful for the preclinical research [4]. Empirical evidences suggest that when these phospholipids are rigorously stirred in the aqueous phase, they form closed configurations and since these structures are hollow, they could easily transport drugs regardless of their nature [5]. Liposomes can restrict cargos from deteriorating in the surrounding biological environment, enhance their bio-distribution and facilitate their administration to the target cells when compared with the conventional naked administration of drugs.

Various types of liposomes exist includes conventional, fusogenic, cationic, long circulatory, pH sensitive and immuno-liposomes that are categorized as per their formulation and composition [6]. The major role of liposomes has been explored in the area of drug delivery for developing interventional approaches against the infectious diseases. Of late, different drug delivery systems comprising of liposomes are approved by WHO and many others are in the process of being approved for translational research. Here, we have summarized a fewer of them that are currently under investigation.

Park *et al.*, has developed anti-HER2 (ErbB2) immuno-liposome loaded with the anticancer drugs for the targeted delivery for the over-expressing HER cancer

IntechOpen

cells [7]. Similarly, a liposomal formulation of cytarabine (DepoCyte®) is developed to treat neoplastic meningitis. The protraction period for neurological development, improved the quality of life and efficacies response rate was observed [8]. Doxil® was the first drug approved by the FDA against cancer [9]. Further, the role of liposomes has also been explored for the parasitic infection of visceral Leishmaniasis by using the formulation of liposome entrapped amphotericin B [10]. Currently, research is ongoing to explore the role of liposomes as biolubricant on artificial joints and promising results were observed which can be enhanced by increasing the length of liposomal carbon chain [11]. Additionally, it has been used for the combinational therapy. Paclitaxal and doxorubicin loaded liposomal formulation provides better therapeutic results compare to that seen with the physical mixture of the drugs with reduced toxic effects of individual drugs [12]. Later on, arginine-glycine-aspartate (R-G-D) based liposomes formulations rendered lesser toxicity and greater tumor inhibition [13]. Furthermore, liposomal amphotericin B along with flucytosine and fluconazole have been used for the treatment of HIV mediated cryptococcal meningitis and found promising as compared to the treatment approved by WHO with fewer adverse events [14]. The detailed information about the role of liposomes in malaria infection and its role for the determining the immunogenicity of candidate antigens aiming at developing vaccines has been reviewed recently [15]. It has been also explored for the current pandemic condition of COVID-19 and its contribution in different vaccine formulations [16].

2. Engineered liposomes: better nanocarriers

Liposomes have been used as a vehicle to deliver the drugs sustainably. However, with time, the advancement in the formulation of liposomes and their engineering helped overcome the associated issues. The composition and characteristics of liposomes differ, based on the technique of formulation, and charge present on their surface. Moreover, selection of bilayer components ultimately influences the sturdiness or fluidity of the formulated vesicles [5]. The bilayer is coupled with hydrophobic compounds and lipid vesicles potentially carry hydrophobic, hydrophilic chemicals or both. The fusion of this bilayer with cell membrane allows the site-specific and targeted administration of drugs or vaccine candidates. Nevertheless, encapsulated content delivery via liposomal formulation is a complex process. The first generation of the liposomes could overcome the problems of stability. Moreover, their composition involves the neutral or negatively charged phospholipid and cholesterol. Hence, the issues associated with the conventional liposomes were addressed by the engineered liposomes using distearoyl-phosphatidylcholine cholesterol and saturated phospholipid [17].

The conventional liposomal formulation methods involve the thin film hydration, reverse phase evaporation, solvent injection and elimination of detergent. One of the most common liposomes preparation procedures is the thin-film method; it operates by forming a thin lipid coating on the inner wall of the rotary evaporator flask. The key benefit of this process is its remarkable reproducibility even when operating with small amounts of compounds. However, lower encapsulation efficiency has been a major drawback of the thin-film method [18]. Another liposomal preparation method (injection method) has many variations and liposome formulation involves the injection of organic solvent (ethanol or ether) dissolved lipids in the aqueous solution [19]. The emulsification or reverse-phase evaporation method is similar to the injection method involving the lipids, dissolved in the organic solvent and combined with both organic and water phase. The main advantage of the emulsification approach is that it offers the higher encapsulation efficiency than that with the injection methods [17]. The use of liposome is for the drug delivery which needs encapsulation of drug. Active and passive methods have been used for the drug encapsulation [20].

3. Liposomes mediated drug delivery

People are heavily dependent upon the use of antibiotics but the antibiotic resistance forced us finding other alternatives. Therefore, liposomes that closely mirror the cell membrane of the host, target bacterial toxins are explored. Moreover, these delivery vehicles have been used in the clinical settings to transport drugs and candidate antigens for their targeted and sustained release [21]. Recently, the ability of liposomes laden with immune stimulatory molecules to enhance the efficacy of cancer immunotherapy has been investigated [22, 23]. Using an antibody-based strategy, immunoliposomes have formulated which are specific to the cancer cells or endothelial cells of the tumor vasculature [24]. The research carried out by Zhang *et al.* showed that usage of PEGylated-immunoliposomes in murine melanoma model has shown the comparable immune-stimulatory activity to the free and with no systemic toxicity [25].

Since, one of the crucial components of the effective cancer immunotherapy is the efficient and selective transport of these stimulating chemicals to the cells of interest. Therefore, utilizing liposomes in immunostimulatory therapy can produce significant anti-tumor effects without causing systemic side effects and hence suggestive of the therapeutic application of liposome loaded drugs.

Enzyme-responsive liposomes are another method for the administration of anticancer drugs for several extracellular enzymes such as secreted phospholipase A2 (sPLA2), matrix metalloproteinases (MMPs), and intracellular enzymes (cathepsin) [26]. According to recent studies, polymeric and PEGylated liposomal nanoparticles (PLNs) can suppress antitumor immunity and promote tumor growth in murine models by preventing PLN-induced tumor growth and improved progression-free survival [27]. Recently, delivery of Bortezomib, a protease inhibitor was used for the treatment of multiple myeloma (MM) when delivered through liposomes in the humanized mouse model for MM has shown the complete tumor regression [28]. It suggests the therapeutic role of drugs mediated by the liposomes in cancer therapy. Besides, humanized mouse developed for the chronic myelomonocytic leukemia (CMML) using the patient-derived induced pluripotent stem cells (iPSCs) has confirmed the role of clodronate drug when used the liposome formulation in CMML therapy [29].

4. Limitations of liposomes as a delivery vehicle

The major hurdle of the liposome is to deal with stability, uptake by liver, spleen and lungs and the short half-life in blood. Liposomes, like any exogenous particle that enters our body, are challenged with several defensive systems, for instance- the reticuloendothelial system (RES), opsonization, and immunogenicity, which are designed to recognize, neutralize and eliminate the invading substances.

Following systemic delivery, RES is the primary location for liposome accumulation followed by liver, spleen, kidney, lungs, bone marrow, and lymph nodes associated with RES. Plasma proteins and liposomal drug delivery systems tend to interact and their degree of interaction is crucial for defining the toxicity, efficacy and bio-distribution. Hence, plasma proteins are significant for RES-mediated opsonization and vesicular instability. Highly charged liposomes are more prone to get eliminated by the liver in minutes and the spleen within an hour.

Our intricate immune system can get triggered by the liposomal systems causing activation of the complement system that leads to the acute hypersensitivity syndrome known as complement activation-related pseudoallergy (CARPA) originating as a multitude of immunological and inflammatory processes. The complement system can be triggered by the varieties of liposomes; however, some specific liposomal characteristics elevate the tendency for complement activation, which include surface charge, absence of liposomal homogeneity, expanding size, endotoxin contamination, presence of ≥70% cholesterol in the bilayer membrane. Thus, neutral compact unimellar vesicles are found to be the poorest reactogenic species of these liposomal systems [4].

Individual variances in the EPR effect, the accelerated blood clearance (ABC) phenomena of PEGylated liposomes, scale-up, reproducibility/consistency among different batches and manufacturing sites, and excipients management is the key challenges throughout the development and commercialization of liposomes [30]. Assessing the pharmacokinetics, pharmacodynamics, and toxicity of a formulation after injection becomes increasingly challenging as the number of physicochemical variables in a nano-formulation preparation rises.

Across several biomedical fields, the application of liposomes to facilitate drug delivery has already had a massive effect. Prospective research will improve the existing liposomal platforms and help understand the current regulatory constraints by gaining a better understanding of the breakthroughs in liposomal technology as well as overcome the impediments.

5. Controlling residual innate immune responses for the sizeable grafting of human cells/tissues

The early development of knock-in/out mice to understand the host-pathogen interaction has paved the way forward. This in turn results into the higher efficacy of vaccine development. However, usage of surrogate models often resulting in the failure of clinical trials for numerous vaccine candidates. To address this issue, the concept of transplanting human cells into immunodeficient mouse which mimics the human-system has emerged and known as 'humanized mouse". Later on, advancement in the technology aided in the generation of mouse-human chimera for various biomedical applications. These mouse human chimeras have responded pretty well to understand the pathogens and their interaction with the host.

Normal or malignant human hematopoietic stem cells (huHSC) were transplanted into immunodeficient mice to develop the humanized mouse model. The success of mouse humanization depends upon the susceptibility of the host immune system towards acceptance of the graft. Therefore, different approaches have been adopted. The use of the liposome loaded with clodronate (clo-lip) drug showed the depletion of the cells of monocyte/macrophages lineage (**Figure 1**). This showed the successful engraftment of huHSC in SCID mice [31]. Further, Hu *et al.*, developed the humanized mouse model (in NOD/SCID or NOD/SCID/γc−/−) having the matured $CD71^{-}CD235a^{+}$ human red blood cells (huRBCs) however their poor efficiency as well as meager number of RBCs makes it difficult to use these mice to study various hematological disorders. Moreover, cobra venom factor (CVF) when combined with clo-lip has shown the extended survival of huRBCs in immunodeficient mice. It could help studying the function of RBCs and human erythropoiesis [32]. Since macrophages have been the major stumbling block resulting in the poor reconstitution of human platelets in human $CD34^{+}$ cells-grafted mice, clo-lip treatment showed the higher level of human platelet in the periphery of chimeric mice [33]. This chimeric mouse has opened a door to study the step-wise development of human thrombopoiesis and function of platelets (**Figure 1**).

Poor understanding of the host-pathogen interaction is the major issue for the successful development of an asexual blood stage vaccine for malaria as well as for developing an understanding of the liver-stage (LS) infection of human malaria. It has been evident that treatment with clo-lip to transgenic/immunodeficient mice (TK/NOG) helped the successful transplantation of human hepatocytes (huHep) that allows the development of exoerythrocytic stages of malaria in murine models [34, 35]. The clo-lip formulation induces the apoptosis and depletes the monocytes-macrophages lineage allowing the sizeable engraftment of huHep in mice liver to develop human live chimeric mouse inevitably required to study LS infection of *P. falciparum*. Further advancements have allowed studying the asexual blood stage and transition from LS to asexual blood stage infection of *P. falciparum* in one host [36]. Similarly, another humanized mouse has developed (HIS-HEry mice) using clo-lip formulation to study of asexual blood stage infection of *Plasmodium vivax* that exhibits erythropoiesis following hematopoietic stem and progenitor cells (HSPCs) transplantation [37] (**Figure 1**).

Having confirmed the role of clo-lip in developing the humanized mouse models, Youssef and colleagues have explored the role of clo-lip in to reduce the skin allograft rejection. Data has shown that intraperitoneal injection of clo-lip markedly reduced the macrophage-lineage and hence conferred the extended survival of skin allograft in CD8 knockout mice as compared to that seen with control [38]. Similarly, clo-lip was seen to treat macrophages activation syndrome (MAS) or haemophagocytic lymphoistiocytosis, a life-threatening condition that leads to the multiple-organ failure (**Figure 1**) [39]. Very recently, role of clo-lip has also been explored in the insect system to study the innate immune response wherein depletion of phagocytic immune cells takes place in *Drosophila melanogaster* and *Aedes aegypti* mosquito [40].

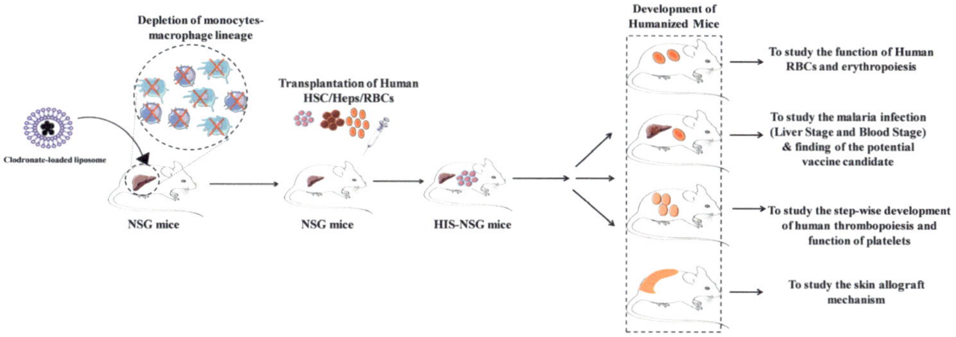

Figure 1.
Controlling residual innate immune response by the clodronate-loaded (clo-lip) liposome for the development of humanized mice. Clo-lip depletes the cells of monocyte-macrophage lineage in the immunodeficient mice (left panel). The human hematopoietic stem cells, hepatocytes or red blood cells were transplanted in these mice and generate the human-immune system mice (HIS-NSG) (middle panel). These HIS-NSG mice are used in the translational biomedical research and vaccine development (right panel).

6. Conclusions

The conventional delivery systems have earned popularity due to their economic, simple and user-friendly approach. However, recently developed specific drug delivery systems such as liposomes attracted the researchers for their target specificity, effectiveness and minimum adverse effects. The effectiveness of treatment is associated with the ability of drug to target and affect the biological functions of ailing cells and rendering minimum damage to the healthy tissues. Liposomes may be composed of one or more lipid bilayer. With the length of phospholipid and the liposome component ratio decide the liposome stability, efficiency and stability which further aid in designing the drug-delivery system for site and target-specific delivery. Further, work on usage of liposomes in the development of humanized mouse model(s) and determination of immunogenic potential of candidate antigens [41–43] has opened vistas to explore their role in translational biomedical research.

Acknowledgements

Rajeev Tyagi would like to express his gratitude to DBT, New Delhi, Ramalingaswami Re-entry Fellowship Project (No. BT/RLF/Re-entry/27/2018) and Indian Council of Medical Research (ICMR), New Delhi extramural grant (35/1/2020-Nano/BMS) for generously supporting this study. Rajeev K. Tyagi would like to express his thanks to the central MIL facility of CSIR-IMTECH, Chandigarh. Nikunj Tandel would like to thank the Nirma University and the Indian Council of Medical Research (ICMR) for providing the fellowship to carry out his research (ICMR award letter No.: 2020-7623/CMB-BMS). The figure has been prepared using Servier Medical ART: SMART (smart.servier.com).

Conflict of interest

The authors declare no conflict of interest.

Abbreviations

Clo-lip	Liposome loaded with clodronate
CMML	Chronic myelomonocytic leukemia
HSPCs	Hematopoietic stem and progenitor cells
huHSC	Human hematopoietic stem cells
huRBCs	Human red blood cells
iPSC	induced pluripotent stem cells
LS	Liver-stage
MM	Multiple myeloma
MMPs	Matrix metalloproteinases
PLNs	PEGylated liposomal nanoparticles
RES	Reticuloendothelial system

Author details

Prakriti Sharma[1†], Mili Mehta[2†], Nikunj Tandel[2] and Rajeev K. Tyagi[1*]

1 Division of Cell Biology and Immunology, Biomedical Parasitology and Nano-Immunology Lab, CSIR-Institute of Microbial Technology (IMTECH), Chandigarh, India

2 Institute of Science, Nirma University, Ahmedabad, Gujarat, India

*Address all correspondence to: rajeevtyagi@imtech.res.in; rajeev.gru@gmail.com

† Co-first authors (contributed equally).

References

[1] Xing H et al. Recent developments of liposomes as Nanocarriers for Theranostic applications. Theranostics. 2016;**6**(9):1336-1352

[2] Bozzuto G, Molinari A. Liposomes as nanomedical devices. International Journal of Nanomedicine. 2015;**10**:975-999

[3] Kim EM, Jeong HJ. Liposomes: Biomedical applications. Chonnam Medical Journal. 2021;**57**(1):27-35

[4] Sercombe L et al. Advances and challenges of liposome assisted drug delivery. Frontiers in Pharmacology. 2015;**6**:286

[5] Wagner A, Vorauer-Uhl K. Liposome technology for industrial purposes. Journal of Drug Delivery. 2011;**2011**:591325

[6] Nakhaei P et al. Liposomes: Structure, biomedical applications, and stability parameters with emphasis on cholesterol. Frontiers in Bioengineering and Biotechnology. 2021;**9**:705886

[7] Park JW et al. Tumor targeting using anti-her2 immunoliposomes. Journal of Controlled Release. 2001;**74**(1-3):95-113

[8] Rueda Domínguez A et al. Liposomal cytarabine (DepoCyte) for the treatment of neoplastic meningitis. Clinical & Translational Oncology. 2005;**7**(6):232-238

[9] Barenholz Y. Doxil®--the first FDA-approved nano-drug: Lessons learned. Journal of Controlled Release. 2012;**160**(2):117-134

[10] Bern C et al. Liposomal amphotericin B for the treatment of visceral leishmaniasis. Clinical Infectious Diseases. 2006;**43**(7):917-924

[11] Wang Z et al. Investigation of the lubrication properties and synergistic interaction of biocompatible liposome-polymer complexes applicable to artificial joints. Colloids and Surfaces. B, Biointerfaces. 2019;**178**:469-478

[12] Yu J et al. Remote loading paclitaxel-doxorubicin prodrug into liposomes for cancer combination therapy. Acta Pharmaceutica Sinica B. 2020;**10**(9):1730-1740

[13] Fu S et al. Integrin α(v)β(3)-targeted liposomal drug delivery system for enhanced lung cancer therapy. Colloids and Surfaces. B, Biointerfaces. 2021;**201**:111623

[14] Jarvis JN et al. Single-dose liposomal amphotericin B treatment for Cryptococcal meningitis. The New England Journal of Medicine. 2022;**386**(12):1109-1120

[15] Memvanga PB, Nkanga CI. Liposomes for malaria management: The evolution from 1980 to 2020. Malaria Journal. 2021;**20**(1):327

[16] Attia MA et al. Brief on recent application of liposomal vaccines for lower respiratory tract viral infections: From influenza to COVID-19 vaccines. Pharmaceuticals (Basel). 2021;**14**(11):1173

[17] Nsairat H et al. Liposomes: Structure, composition, types, and clinical applications. Heliyon. 2022;**8**(5):e09394

[18] Šturm L, Poklar Ulrih N. Basic methods for preparation of liposomes and studying their interactions with

different compounds, with the emphasis on polyphenols. International Journal of Molecular Sciences. 2021;**22**(12):6547

[19] William B et al. Supercritical fluid methods: An alternative to conventional methods to prepare liposomes. Chemical Engineering Journal. 2020;**383**:123106

[20] Pattni BS et al. New developments in liposomal drug delivery. Chemical Reviews. 2015;**115**(19):10938-10966

[21] Henry BD et al. Engineered liposomes sequester bacterial exotoxins and protect from severe invasive infections in mice. Nature Biotechnology. 2015;**33**(1):81-88

[22] Rueda F et al. Effect of TLR ligands co-encapsulated with multiepitopic antigen in nanoliposomes targeted to human DCs via fc receptor for cancer vaccines. Immunobiology. 2017;**222**(11):989-997

[23] Cruz LJ et al. Liposomes containing NY-ESO-1/tetanus toxoid and adjuvant peptides targeted to human dendritic cells via the fc receptor for cancer vaccines. Nanomedicine (London, England). 2014;**9**(4):435-449

[24] Kunjachan S et al. Noninvasive imaging of nanomedicines and Nanotheranostics: Principles, Progress, and prospects. Chemical Reviews. 2015;**115**(19):10907-10937

[25] Zhang Y et al. Nanoparticle anchoring targets immune agonists to tumors enabling anti-cancer immunity without systemic toxicity. Nature Communications. 2018;**9**(1):6

[26] Olusanya TOB et al. Liposomal drug delivery systems and anticancer drugs. Molecules. 2018;**23**(4):907

[27] Rajan R et al. Liposome-induced immunosuppression and tumor growth is mediated by macrophages and mitigated by liposome-encapsulated alendronate. Journal of Controlled Release. 2018;**271**:139-148

[28] Deshantri AK et al. Complete tumor regression by liposomal Bortezomib in a humanized mouse model of multiple myeloma. Hema. 2020;**4**(5):e463

[29] Taoka K et al. Using patient-derived iPSCs to develop humanized mouse models for chronic myelomonocytic leukemia and therapeutic drug identification, including liposomal clodronate. Scientific Reports. 2018;**8**(1):15855

[30] Liu P et al. A review of liposomes as a drug delivery system: Current status of approved products, regulatory environments, and future perspectives. Molecules. 2022;**27**(4):1372

[31] Terpstra W et al. Facilitated engraftment of human hematopoietic cells in severe combined immunodeficient mice following a single injection of Cl2MDP liposomes. Leukemia. 1997;**11**(7):1049-1054

[32] Chen B et al. Complement depletion improves human red blood cell reconstitution in Immunodeficient mice. Stem Cell Reports. 2017;**9**(4):1034-1042

[33] Hu Z, Yang YG. Full reconstitution of human platelets in humanized mice after macrophage depletion. Blood. 2012;**120**(8):1713-1716

[34] Arnold L et al. Further improvements of the P. falciparum humanized mouse model. PLoS One. 2011;**6**(3):e18045

[35] Arnold L et al. Analysis of innate defences against plasmodium falciparum in immunodeficient mice. Malaria Journal. 2010;**9**:197

[36] Tyagi RK et al. Humanized mice are instrumental to the study of plasmodium falciparum infection. Frontiers in Immunology. 2018;**9**:2550

[37] Luiza-Batista C et al. Humanized mice for investigating sustained plasmodium vivax blood-stage infections and transmission. Nature Communications. 2022;**13**(1):4123

[38] Youssef A-R. The effect of in vivo macrophage depletion on skin allograft rejection in wild-type and CD8 knockout mice. Turkish Journal of Immunology. 2020;**8**(2):57-64

[39] Nishiwaki S et al. In vivo tracking of transplanted macrophages with near infrared fluorescent dye reveals temporal distribution and specific homing in the liver that can be perturbed by clodronate liposomes. PLoS One. 2020;**15**(12):e0242488

[40] Ramesh Kumar J et al. Use of Clodronate liposomes to deplete phagocytic immune cells in Drosophila melanogaster and Aedes aegypti. Frontiers in Cell and Development Biology. 2021;**9**:627976

[41] Marepally S et al. Editorial: Nanomedicine in infectious diseases: Drug delivery and vaccines. Frontiers in Pharmacology. 2022;**13**:928572

[42] Chaudhari R et al. Transdermal immunization of elastic liposome-laden recombinant chimeric fusion protein of P. falciparum (PfMSP-Fu(24)) mounts protective immune response. Nanomaterials (Basel). 2021;**11**(2):406

[43] Tyagi RK et al. Elastic liposome-mediated transdermal immunization enhanced the immunogenicity of P. falciparum surface antigen, MSP-119. Vaccine. 2015;**33**(36):4630-4638

Chapter 2

Liposomal Nanoparticles: A Viable Nanoscale Drug Carriers for the Treatment of Cancer

Bunty Sharma, Sampan Attri, Jyoti Syal and Ujjawal Sharma

Abstract

Cancer immunotherapy is emerging as a promising therapeutic modality for achieving highly efficient therapeutic performance while avoiding tumor metastasis and relapse which are most common outcome of traditional cancer therapies (surgery, chemo and radiotherapy). Liposomal nanoparticles may be an ideal platform for systemic immune modulator delivery. Liposomes, the lipid bilayer vesicles, are biocompatible biodegradable carriers that are extensively used for the delivery of both hydrophilic and hydrophobic bio actives. The advance features like structural fabrication of liposome for ligand anchoring, long-circulation, and stimuli-responsiveness are helpful for the demand of clinical and industrial uses. Recent studies have reported the manifestations of liposomal newer developments in cancer treatment. Presentchapter discusses the most recent advances in liposomal nanoparticles for cancer therapy along with ligand targeted, stimulus targeted and autophagy modulation by liposomal nanoparticles for cancer treatment.

Keywords: liposomes, nanoparticles, cancer, treatment, drug delivery

1. Introduction

Cancer is a huge and enormous health challenge of the current century, in which the active cells of body become abnormal and multiply at uncontrollable rate. The major cause for this disease is environmental toxins which further damage the DNA structure. As per the report of World Health Organization (WHO) 2018, cancer is the second most leading cause of deaths around the world. Approximately 9.5 million people had died due to different types of cancers in a year. A continuous increasing in new patients and mortality rate due to cancer clearly indicates that there is an urgent need for the development of new techniques for its treatment. One of the effective and major treatments of cancer is chemotherapy with anticarcinogenic agents. But due to lack of appropriate sensitivity and specificity, chemotherapy with anticarcinogenic agents is ineffective. Also, this method of treatment of the cancer has been restricted due to its ill effects [1].

There are various traditional medicines which show poor materiamedica, restricted pharmacokinetics and deadly toxins, which administered controlled use

 IntechOpen

of these drugs. To deal with these problems and upgrade the remedial indexes of the medicine, the emerging fields of nanotechnology and nanomedicine have made denoting development in disclosure, interpretation and medication of numerous diseases at the initial level [2]. In the current scenario, use of liposomes nanoparticles has made it feasible to reduce the toxicity and enhance the pharmacology parameters, such as delivery, extended transmission time, focused composed discharge, increased intracellular concentration, upgraded solvency and stability of drugs in the living being. All these important points have been attained by using the delivery systems of medicines with nanoparticles ranging from 1 to 100 nm diameter, where a huge facet results in expanded cellular communication and numerous modifications of facet attributes. Further, by rendering various medicines, medication using nanoparticles have also facilitated synergetic treatments and refrained medicine protection [3].

Present article is an attempt to summarize the findings of the exploration and fabrication of liposomes and various attributes of liposomes. An attempt has also made to analyze the availability and development of liposomal medicines, being used for cancer treatment in the market. Eventually, a report related to fortuities and disputes related to the utilization of nanomedicines related to liposomes will be deduced, that can be used to highlight it as a crucial issue for the future research of the scientists. The result of it can be the abolition of the restrictions and nourishing the beneficial points. They represent an expansive extent of clinical stage nanotherapeutics because of their degradable, compatible, non-poisonous, and insusceptible formation. The amphiphobic phosphatide layer of liposomes are almost similar to the marsupial cell layer which enables a systematic interaction between nanoparticles and cell layer. In this way, it enhances the feasible cellular intake. Moreover, these nanoparticles may be included with molecules for extended productivity and particularly selecting injured cells. This improves pharmacological medicine of liposome and their capacity to traverse target cells, coming to absorption of interior cells, thus, reducing toxicants and enhancing medication viability. Liposome embodiment may decrease sedate endorsement by the immune and excretory organ, thus increasing transmission period in the blood and enhancing their accessibility [4]. Another profit of nanoparticles in their thermo heat sensitive aspect, i.e., arise of degrees (40–41°C) in packing leads to changes in the bilayer, which soothes the discharge of the encapsulated medicine. These thermo-devices favor the discharge of a great amount of the anticancer drug to a heat-treated location in the tumor, when an external source of heat is used, thus keeping away the harm to the bordering normal tissue [5].

2. Liposomes mediated delivery of anticancer drugs

Liposomes are dual layered spherical cells which include saturated fats and cholesterol. They create a minimum of one lipoid dual layer in water, surrounding a liquid base that may enclose both hydrophilic medicines and hydrophobic compounds submerged via means of lamellae by Van der Waals. Phospholipids are amphipathic liquids that include glycerol molecules certain to a group of phosphate (PO_4^{2-}) and dual chains of fatty acid which can be moistened or un-moistened. The phosphate has also a close bondage with an organic particle, e.g., mono-ethanolamine or choline. Lecithins are key ingredients which provide distinctive features to liposomes, such as how the compounds are encapsulated and how they function inside the body. Both liposomal and plasmalemma can coincide during the release operation as phospholipids are the main biological components of tissue membrane [6].

3. History of liposomes

The discovery of the cell by Anthony Van Hook in the late seventeenth century prompted a lot of questions about how cells are formed. The presence of phospholipid dual layers in plasma layers was discovered by Ten, Gorter and Grendel in 1925. Later, the dual layers clutter layer model was later described by Singer and Nicolson to explain the behavior of plasma layers phospholipids. These research-based studies and hypothesis captivated the attention of other scientists to nanoparticles derived from fats. Then, it was in 1965 when Alec D. Bangham discovered liposomes and were named as "banghosomes". Later, "banghosomes" were renamed by Gerald Weissmann as liposomes in 1968. Liposomes belonged to such class of therapeutic nanoparticles used in cancer treatment which was the first to get approval worldwide [7].

4. Size and structure of liposomes

The diameter of liposomes starts from 20 nm to greater than numerous hundred micrometers. The size of the particle affects their material medica, tissue extravasations, dispersal of tissue, hepatic cirrhosis, elimination from kidney, and rate of dispensation from the location of injection. Liposomes of an average diameter ranging from 100 to 150 nm can enter into the liver epidermis, subordinate formation of lymphoids, or the contexture of tumors. As it were liposomes with one of these breadths which can simply elude from blood arteries that pervade tissues, e.g. heart, lung and kidney. In contrast, molecules having diameter lower than 10 nm may filter via the glomerular artery and may not re-assimilate. It can be noted that liposomes with a diameter of 100–150 nm are the most important for cell uptake. As the liposome diameter is decreased to 50 nm or less greatly decreases dispensation of endocytosis, so the system endocytosis is also particularly important. Thus, the liposomes which are within the range of 50 nm –100 nm, keep away endocytosis and take extended blood transmission time. Subsequently, the ideal range size of liposomes ranges between 80 and 150 nm [8].

Liposomes basically consist of phospholipids. Phosphatides are a form of liquids, which are in similarity with triglycerides. There is a pillar of difluoride and two chains of hydrophobic in the formation of Phosphatides. In this way Phosphatides are considered amphiphilic atoms (**Figure 1**).

Phospholipids liposome membrane mainly contain phosphatidylcholine, phosphatidylethanolamine, phosphatidylserine, and sphingomyelin which are amphiphilic in nature and have a strong propensity to create specific configuration in water.

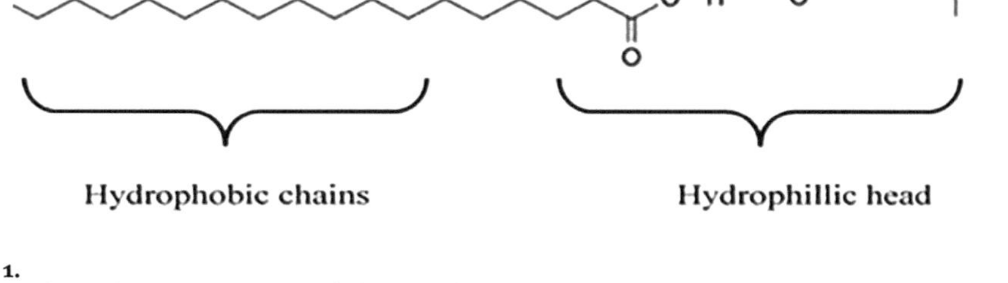

Figure 1.
The non-polar and polar components of Phosphatides.

The primary cause of this appearance is that phospholipids include two hydrophobic tails (fatty acids) and a hydrophilic head (phosphate molecule). The phosphate group gather interatomic with H_2O polar atoms, whereas the hydrophobic tails elude from water atoms and interact with each other.

5. Classification of liposome

The size, number of phospholipid bilayers, mix method, and production procedure of liposomes can all be used to classify them. Liposomes can be categorized into three sizes: tiny, medium, and giant, based on their size. Vesicles can be unilamellar, oligolamellar, or multilamellar, depending on the number of membrane layers. In this respect, it can be stated that the unilamellar vesicles are phospholipid bilayer-containing liposomes that range in size from 50 to 250 nm, whereas multilamellar vesicles are much bigger, approximately 0.5–1.5 μm, and also comprise various phospholipid bilayer membranes. Diverse liposomes have definite system of preparation. In the majority of these production techniques, lipids are solved in order to produce liposome membranes using a specific solvent (such as methanol, chloroform etc.). Other techniques for producing liposomes include French pressure cells, sonication, reverse phase evaporation, freeze-drying and membrane extrusion [9].

6. Therapeutic applications of liposomes

In comparison to the existing formulations, liposomes provide superior therapeutic efficacy and safety [10]. Some of the main the remedial implementation of liposomes in the delivery of remedial medicines include:

6.1 Site-avoidance drug delivery

The cytotoxicity of anti-angiogenic medicines of cancer is credited to their narrow remedial index. By decreasing the delivery of medicine to normal cells and by enclosing it in liposomes, the remedial index can be enhanced. For example, doxorubicin has a severe side effect of toxicity related to heart, but when composed as liposomes, the poisonous quality is minimized without any alteration in the therapeutic activity [11].

6.2 Target specific drug delivery

Delivery of a larger fragment of the medicine to the location of tumor/cancer, can be achieved by particular targeting of the location, thereby reducing the drug's exposure to normal tissues. On systemic management, it was found that the expanded circulation of immunoliposomes can recognize and hold together the target membranes with greater accuracy. For example, in patients with repetitive osteogenic sarcoma, an enhanced tumoricidal activity of white blood cells was observed when muramyl peptide derivatives were formulated as liposomes and managed systemically [12].

6.3 Intracellular drug delivery

Enhanced delivery of prospective medicines to the cytoplasm, where sedate receptors are present, can be achieved by utilizing liposome sedate conveyance framework.

Generally, N-(phosphonacetyl)-L-aspartate) is ineffectively taken up into cells. Such drugs when enclosed within liposomes, showed greater action against ovarian tumor cell lines as compared to free drug [13].

6.4 Drug delivery with sustained release

Liposomes produce maintained discharge of target medicines to accomplish the maximum remedial efficiency, which requires an extended plasma concentration at remedial levels. Medicines such as cytosine Arabinoside can be enclosed in liposomes for continuous liberation and improved ejection rate in living organism [14].

6.5 Intraperitoneal administration

Cancer which develops in the spinal cavity can be cured by regulating the medicine to spinal cavity. Nevertheless, the swift dispensation of the medicines from the intra-peritoneal cavity results in decreased quantity of medicine at the infected location. Medicines enclosing liposomes have lower acceptance rates than free medications, and they can deliver the maximum amount of medication in a prolonged manner to the affected area [15].

6.6 Vaccine immunological adjuvants

Liposomes can be utilized to improve the response of immune system by compressing the supplements. Depending on an antigen's lipophilicity, they can be accommodated by liposome in the liquid cavity or assimilate with the dual layers. Liposomes were used for the first time as immunological adjuvants, to increase the immune response of diphtheria toxoid [16].

7. Mechanism of action of liposome

A liposome contains a particular place inside a lipid hydrophobic cell. Hydrophobic substances are easily diluted with the lipid membranes. In this manner, hydrophilic and hydrophobic molecules both are carried by liposomes. Subsequently, the drug's placement will rely on its biophysical characteristics and lipid structure. The lipid bilayers combine with other bilayers of the cell membrane to deliver necessary drug molecules to the site of activity, thereby releasing the liposomal content [17, 18]. Following are the steps which are involved in liposome action of drug delivery:

7.1 Absorption

Absorption of liposomes to layers of cell are the reason of its contact on the layer of the cell.

7.2 Endocytosis

Absorption of liposomes on the surface of the layer of the cell followed by swallowing and internalizing them into the liposomes.

7.3 Combination

Direct transport of the contents of liposomes into the cytoplasm is achieved by combining the lipid dual layers of liposomes with the lipoidal cell membrane by lateral diffusion and mixing of lipids.

7.4 Exchange of lipid

Lipid transfer proteins in the cell membrane quickly recognize liposomes and start lipid exchange because the phospholipids in the liposomal lipid membrane and those in the cell membrane are identical. For instance, cancer cells absorb a large amount of fat to meet the requirement of rapid development. They perceive the anti-cancer drug-loaded liposomes as a potential nutritional source. They are submerged when a liposome focuses on them. When the anti-cancer medications are released from the liposome into the area, the medication starts to kill cancer cells [19].

8. Liposomal formulations for treatment of cancer

The following are the most current clinical results using different liposomal drugs to treat different solid tumors:

8.1 Daunorubicin and doxorubicin

Doxil® is the trademark for the primary PEGylated Liposome Technology medication delivery technology. It comprises doxorubicin hydrochloride, an anthracycline-family anticancer drug that is capsuled. It helps cancer cells undergo caspase-dependent apoptosis brought on by oxidative DNA damage. It inhibits topoisomerase II, an enzyme necessary for the division and growth of cancer cells. Free radicals, reactive oxygen species that can harm membrane structure and result in lipid peroxidation, are also produced by this enzyme [20].

8.2 Paclitaxel and docetaxel

Paclitaxel inhibits the growth of tumor endothelial cells when combined with beta microtubules. As paclitaxel is insoluble in water, therefore, dehydrated ethanol and polyethoxylated castor oil in a 1:1 (v/v) ratio are utilized as preparation instruments, despite the fact that it causes harmful side effects such neuro adulteration, hyperlipemia, and hypersensitivity reactions. Several cremophor-free liposomal paclitaxel (LPTX) synthesis has been permitted by FDA to avoid these drawbacks. Some of the examples include: (i) LEP-ETU, a traditional anionic nanoparticle with an estimate of about 150 nm (ii) EndoTAG™, a cationic liposome structure of lipoid-submerged with chemotherapy drug, which links with negatively charged cells of tumor endocardium reducing the blood supply of the tumor and (iii) Lipusu® a formulation prepared by utilizing film scattering strategies followed by a lyophilization method. Formulations resembling liposomes without the cremophor, such as Genexol-PM, a low-density lipoprotein receptor-binding nanocomposite amphiphilic structure of paclitaxel and PTX-LDE, nanoparticle with lipid core compressed with paclitaxel, which accumulates in the tumor tissues [21].

8.3 Docetaxel

Docetaxel, which is a polymerized taxane equivalent and an antimitotic medium, joinsitself to the beta tubulin. It is also the reason of stabilization of tubulin polymerization. This stabilization prevents mitosis by breaking microtubules and capturing the G2/M phase of cell cycle. It is frequently used in the treatment of a number of solid tumors but is ineffective in water. The docetaxel (Taxotere) that is now on the market is prepared in ethanol and Tween 80 since it is insoluble in water. However, this substance has been linked to fluid retention over time, severe hypersensitivity reactions, and infusion-related toxicity. To prevent such unfavorable side effects, a number of free Tween 80 and ethanol delivery technologies, including polymeric micelles, nanosomes, nanospheres and protein, have been created and clinically tested [22].

8.4 Mifamurtide

The European Union, Switzerland, and other nations have approved Mepact®, also known as liposomal mifamurtide formulation (liposomal muramyl tripeptide phosphatidylethanolamine), for the treatment of osteosarcoma [23].

8.5 Vincristine

To overcome the dosage, pharmacokinetic, and pharmacodynamic restrictions of non-liposomal vincristine, vincristine sulphate, a semi-synthetic chemotherapeutic drug, has been compressed in sphingomyelin/cholesterol nanoliposomes. Due to its demonstrated safety, the FDA has authorized Marqibo® (Vincristine injection dosage form). Additionally, it demonstrated tolerance as well as improved mononuclear phagocyte system-associated tissues and organs, such as non-Hodgkin lymphomas, vincristine cell uptake, penetration, and concentration [24].

8.6 Cytarabine

Cytarabine is available in a slow-release dose form called liposomal cytarabine (Depocyt®), which causes cytotoxic quantities of the drug to last for at least a week in the cerebrospinal fluid. However, non-liposomal cytarabine is only sustained for 24 hours. When used under supervision as first-line therapy and in conjunction with dexamethasone, Depocyt ® has acceptable toxicity. All of this strongly suggests that it might be crucial in the future for enhancing outcomes for kids with acute lymphoblastic leukemia [14].

9. Engineered tumor target liposomes

In view of its potential for safety and efficacy for site-specific medication administration, liposomes are regarded as the model biomembranes. Cancer has a complicated microenvironment, thus developing tumor-targeted liposomes that include features like remote control or tumor stimuli response to promote tumor extravasation and specific ligands for efficient intracellular localization within tumor cells is necessary [25]. Acute myelogenous leukemia has been treated with folate-anchored Dox-loaded liposomes following all-trans retinoic acid stimulation of folate receptors [26]. A peptide analogue of ApoE3 targeted to low density lipoprotein receptor made it easier to penetrate the blood–brain barrier for dual targeting using distinct ligands, which improved the targeting capabilities of transferrin MAb functionalized liposomes [27]. The PC-3 tumor cells (a prostate cancer cell line) showed observable cellular accumulation in response to the RPARPAR liposomes loaded with doxorubicin, which resulted in greater tumor growth suppression [28]. Multidrug resistance mechanism may not apply to engineered liposomes (due to Pglycoproteins that pump out doxorubicin or vincristine) [29]. By using pH-, temperature-, or photosensitive engineered liposomes, also known as stimuli responsive liposomes, to trigger or control drug release upon effective tumor microenvironment utilization, it is possible to ensure higher accrual of such multidrug-resistant/susceptible drugs after their internalization into target cells [30]. When compared to a control liposome, those loaded with Doxorubicin and Magnevist (a magnetic resonance imaging agent) and anchored with hyaluronic acid-ceramide demonstrated greater cell uptake as a result of the interaction between hyaluronic acid and CD44 receptors. Tagalakis et al. [31] reported serum-stable PEGylated liposomes coupled with peptide for the transfection of plasmid DNA and found that PEGylation increased self-assembly and cell uptake by receptor-mediated endocytosis. Gao et al. [32] focused their work on the characterization, therapeutic effectiveness, advances in antibody engineering, and potential applications of monoclonal antibody-anchored liposomes for cancer chemotherapy. PEGylated immunoliposomes with anti-human epidermal growth factor receptor antibodies, like cetuximab, accumulated more in glioblastoma multiforme [33]. Noble et al., [34] provided a thorough analysis of the challenges presented by modified liposomes for the treatment of cancer, including quicker blood clearance, queered targeting caused by RES absorption, and poor tumor penetrability. Dequalinium and epirubicin-loaded liposomes with a positive charge showed increased cytotoxicity in vitro and anticancer effectiveness in animals [35]. Similar to this, dequalinium displayed efficient mitochondrial targeting in topotecan-loaded liposomes, enhancing therapeutic efficacy in vivo in comparison to untargeted liposomes [36]. Triphenyl-phosphonium, a mitocancerotropic drug, and folic acid coupling to DOX-loaded liposomes have both been shown to improve tumor targeting potential through greater accumulation in mitochondria [37].

10. Conclusions and future perspectives

Since its discovery in 1964, liposomes have a broader range of applications. Whether they are man-made or naturally occurring, the lipids that make up liposomes each have different uses, benefits, and drawbacks. Traditional pharmaceuticals must pass through numerous obstructions and hostile environments in the body that degrade them in order to reach the desired location, including the blood brain barrier, the intestinal wall barrier, the liver, the bloodstream's proteins and enzymes, and the stomach's acidity. Pharmacological substances in the form of liposomes can travel through the body and act as a means of transport to get to the desired tissue, organ, or receptor. Phosphatidyl-choline is the most widely utilized lipid component due to its neutrality and affordability. As previously mentioned, studies have shown that encapsulating anticancer medications like daunorubicin, doxorubicin, and cytarabine in liposomes has therapeutic advantages.

Liposomes can be categorized based on their size, shape, composition, and manufacturing procedure. Greater therapeutic effectiveness against infections, enhanced drug-target selectivity, and improved pharmacokinetics and pharmacodynamics are all advantages of employing liposomes as a drug delivery vehicle. On the other hand, the disadvantages include problems with stability and short shelf-life, problems with encapsulation effectiveness, and problems with sterilization. Certain lipids, particularly charged lipids, become poisonous in increasing concentrations. However, if a therapeutic drug is consumed in excess of a particular amount, it may turn toxic and seriously harm one or more body organs. As a result, the liposome formulation needs to be carefully and effectively created. Future research will be able to improve on existing platforms and solve the current translational and regulatory limits by having a better understanding of the advancements in liposomal technology to date and the hurdles that still need to be overcome. The way liposomes interact with cells affects how well a medicine is delivered. In recent years, liposomes have been used as drug delivery vehicles with a few commercially available formulations that demonstrate increased effectiveness. For further translational success, it will be necessary for professionals involved in manufacturing, pharmaceutical design, cellular interactions and toxicology, as well as preclinical and clinical evaluation, to communicate with one another and work together. According to scientific evidence, medicine delivery via liposomes has a bright future.

Conflict of interest

The authors declare no conflict of interest.

Author details

Bunty Sharma[1], Sampan Attri[2], Jyoti Syal[3] and Ujjawal Sharma[4]*

1 Department of Biotechnology, MMEC, Maharishi Markandeshwar (Deemed to Be University), Ambala, India

2 Viral Testing Facility, Forensic Science Laboratory, Mohali, India

3 Department of Humanities, MMEC, Maharishi Markandeshwar (Deemed to Be University), Ambala, India

4 Department of Human Genetics and Molecular Medicine, School of Health Sciences, Central University of Punjab, Bathinda, India

*Address all correspondence to: ujjawalbiotech@gmail.com

References

[1] Mattiuzzi C, Lippi G. Current cancer epidemiology. Journal of Epidemiology and Global Health. 2019;**9**(4):217-222. DOI: 10.2991/jegh.k.191008.001

[2] Signorell RD, Luciani P, Brambilla D, Leroux JC. Pharmacokinetics of lipid-drug conjugates loaded into liposomes. European Journal of Pharmaceutics and Biopharmaceutics. 2018;**128**:188-199. DOI: 10.1016/j.ejpb.2018.04.003

[3] Gonda A, Kabagwira J, Senthil GN, Wall NR. Internalization of exosomes through receptor-mediated endocytosis. Molecular Cancer Research. 2019;**17**(2):337-347. DOI: 10.1158/1541-7786.MCR-18-0891

[4] Allen TM, Cullis PR. Liposomal drug delivery systems: From concept to clinical applications. Advanced Drug Delivery Reviews. 2013;**65**(1):36-48. DOI: 10.1016/j.addr.2012.09.037

[5] Nardecchia S, Sánchez-Moreno P, Vicente J, Marchal JA, Boulaiz H. Clinical trials of thermosensitive nanomaterials: An overview. Nanomaterials. 2019;**9**(2):191. DOI: 10.3390/nano9020191

[6] Wang J, Gong J, Wei Z. Strategies for liposome drug delivery systems to improve tumor treatment efficacy. AAPS PharmSciTech. 2021;**23**(1):27. DOI: 10.1208/s12249-021-02179-4

[7] Weissig V. Liposomes came first: The early history of liposomology. Methods in Molecular Biology. 2017;**1522**:1-15. DOI: 10.1007/978-1-4939-6591-5_1

[8] Zamani P, Momtazi-Borojeni AA, Nik ME, Oskuee RK, Sahebkar A. Nanoliposomes as the adjuvant delivery systems in cancer immunotherapy. Journal of Cellular Physiology. 2018;**233**(7):5189-5199. DOI: 10.1002/jcp.26361

[9] Akbarzadeh A, Rezaei-Sadabady R, Davaran S, Joo SW, Zarghami N, Hanifehpour Y, et al. Liposome: Classification, preparation, and applications. Nanoscale Research Letters. 2013;**8**(1):102. DOI: 10.1186/1556-276X-8-102

[10] Daraee H, Etemadi A, Kouhi M, Alimirzalu S, Akbarzadeh A. Application of liposomes in medicine and drug delivery. Artificial Cells, Nanomedicine, and Biotechnology. 2016;**44**(1):381-391. DOI: 10.3109/21691401.2014.953633

[11] Rommasi F, Esfandiari N. Liposomal nanomedicine: Applications for drug delivery in cancer therapy. Nanoscale Research Letters. 2021;**16**(1):95. DOI: 10.1186/s11671-021-03553-8

[12] Pillai G. Nanotechnology toward treating cancer: A comprehensive review. In: Applications of Targeted Nano Drugs and Delivery Systems. 2019. pp. 221-256

[13] Unger MM, Wahl J, Ushmorov A, Buechele B, Simmet T, Debatin KM, et al. Enriching suicide gene bearing tumor cells for an increased bystander effect. Cancer Gene Therapy. 2007;**14**(1):30-38. DOI: 10.1038/sj.cgt.7700995

[14] Salehi B, Selamoglu Z, Mileski SK, Pezzani R, Redaelli M, Cho WC, et al. Liposomal cytarabine as cancer therapy: From chemistry to medicine. Biomolecules. 2019;**9**(12):773. DOI: 10.3390/biom9120773

[15] Parker RJ, Hartman KD, Sieber SM. Lymphatic absorption and tissue disposition of liposome-entrapped [14C]

adriamycin following intraperitoneal administration to rats. Cancer Research. 1981;**41**(4):1311-1317

[16] Gregoriadis G, Gursel I, Gursel M, McCormack B. Liposomes as immunological adjuvants and vaccine carriers. Journal of Controlled Release. 1996;**41**(1-2):49-56

[17] Bozzuto G, Molinari A. Liposomes as nanomedical devices. International Journal of Nanomedicine. 2015;**10**:975-999. DOI: 10.2147/IJN.S68861

[18] Liu C, Zhang L, Zhu W, Guo R, Sun H, Chen X, et al. Barriers and strategies of cationic liposomes for cancer gene therapy. Molecular Therapy — Methods & Clinical Development. 2020;**18**:751-764. DOI: 10.1016/j.omtm.2020.07.015

[19] Taft D, Yuan X. Strategies for delivery of cancer chemotherapy. In: Advanced Drug Formulation Design to Optimize Therapeutic Outcomes. Florida, USA: CRC Press; 2007. pp. 191-236

[20] Alavi M, Varma RS. Overview of novel strategies for the delivery of anthracyclines to cancer cells by liposomal and polymeric nanoformulations. International Journal of Biological Macromolecules. 2020;**164**:2197-2203. DOI: 10.1016/j.ijbiomac.2020.07.274

[21] Frederiks CN, Lam SW, Guchelaar HJ, Boven E. Genetic polymorphisms and paclitaxel- or docetaxel-induced toxicities: A systematic review. Cancer Treatment Reviews. 2015;**41**(10):935-950. DOI: 10.1016/j.ctrv.2015.10.010

[22] Razak SAA, Mohd Gazzali A, Fisol FA, Abdulbaqi IM, Parumasivam T, Mohtar N, et al. Advances in nanocarriers for effective delivery of docetaxel in the treatment of lung cancer: An overview. Cancers. 2021;**13**(3):400. DOI: 10.3390/cancers13030400

[23] Biteau K, Guiho R, Chatelais M, Taurelle J, Chesneau J, Corradini N, et al. L-MTP-PE and zoledronic acid combination in osteosarcoma: preclinical evidence of positive therapeutic combination for clinical transfer. American Journal of Cancer Research. 2016;**6**(3):677-689

[24] Wang X, Song Y, Su Y, Tian Q, Li B, Quan J, et al. Are PEGylated liposomes better than conventional liposomes? A special case for vincristine. Drug Delivery. 2016;**23**(4):1092-1100. DOI: 10.3109/10717544.2015.1027015

[25] Jain A, Jain. Advances in tumor targeted liposomes. Current Molecular Medicine. 2018;**18**(1):44-57. DOI: 10.2174/1566524018666180416101522

[26] Torchilin VP. Multifunctional nanocarriers. Advanced Drug Delivery Reviews. 2006;**58**(14):1532-1555. DOI: 10.1016/j.addr.2006.09.009

[27] Markoutsa E, Papadia K, Giannou AD, Spella M, Cagnotto A, Salmona M, et al. Mono and dually decorated nanoliposomes for brain targeting, in vitro and in vivo studies. Pharmaceutical Research. 2014;**31**(5):1275-1289. DOI: 10.1007/s11095-013-1249-3

[28] Yan Z, Yang Y, Wei X, Zhong J, Wei D, Liu L, et al. Tumor-penetrating peptide mediation: An effective strategy for improving the transport of liposomes in tumor tissue. Molecular Pharmaceutics. 2014;**11**(1):218-225. DOI: 10.1021/mp400393a

[29] Jain SK, Jain A. Ligand mediated drug targeted liposomes. In: Liposomal

Delivery Systems: Advances and Challenges. Future Science Book Series. London, UK: Future Science Ltd; 2016. pp. 144-158

[30] Lee SM, Nguyen ST. Smart nanoscale drug delivery platforms from stimuli-responsive polymers and liposomes. Macromolecules. 2013;**46**(23):9169-9180. DOI: 10.1021/ma401529w

[31] Tagalakis AD, Kenny GD, Bienemann AS, McCarthy D, Munye MM, Taylor H, et al. PEGylation improves the receptor-mediated transfection efficiency of peptide-targeted, self-assembling, anionic nanocomplexes. Journal of Controlled Release. 2014;**174**:177-187. DOI: 10.1016/j.jconrel.2013.11.014

[32] Gao J, Chen H, Song H, Su X, Niu F, Li W, et al. Antibody-targeted immunoliposomes for cancer treatment. Mini Reviews in Medicinal Chemistry. 2013;**13**(14):2026-2035. DOI: 10.2174/1389557513666131119202717

[33] Mortensen JH, Jeppesen M, Pilgaard L, Agger R, Duroux M, Zachar V, et al. Targeted antiepidermal growth factor receptor (cetuximab) immunoliposomes enhance cellular uptake in vitro and exhibit increased accumulation in an intracranial model of glioblastoma multiforme. Journal of Drug Delivery. 2013;**2013**:209205. DOI: 10.1155/2013/209205

[34] Noble GT, Stefanick JF, Ashley JD, Kiziltepe T, Bilgicer B. Ligand-targeted liposome design: challenges and fundamental considerations. Trends in Biotechnology. 2014;**32**(1):32-45. DOI: 10.1016/j.tibtech.2013.09.007

[35] Men Y, Wang XX, Li RJ, Zhang Y, Tian W, Yao HJ, et al. The efficacy of mitochondrial targeting antiresistant epirubicin liposomes in treating resistant leukemia in animals. International Journal of Nanomedicine. 2011;**6**: 3125-3137. DOI: 10.2147/IJN.S24847

[36] Weiss MJ, Wong JR, Ha CS, Bleday R, Salem RR, Steele GD Jr, et al. Dequalinium, a topical antimicrobial agent, displays anticarcinoma activity based on selective mitochondrial accumulation. Proceedings of the National Academy of Sciences of the United States of America. 1987;**84**(15):5444-5448. DOI: 10.1073/pnas.84.15.5444

[37] Malhi SS, Budhiraja A, Arora S, Chaudhari KR, Nepali K, Kumar R, et al. Intracellular delivery of redox cycler-doxorubicin to the mitochondria of cancer cell by folate receptor targeted mitocancerotropic liposomes. International Journal of Pharmaceutics. 2012;**432**(1-2):63-74. DOI: 10.1016/j.ijpharm.2012.04.030

Chapter 3

Perspective Chapter: Magnetoliposomes - A Recent Development as Recent Advances in the Field of Controlled Release Drug Delivery

Edyta Maroń, Paweł Krysiński and Michał Chudy

Abstract

The authors of this chapter point out that, although liposomal vesicles are widely used in cancer drug delivery systems, their limitations are also known. Therefore, more recently, new developments in modifications of liposomes have rapidly appeared to improve their parameters, including the maintenance of drugs in their structure, accumulation in target sites, and the active mechanism of drug release. Research on the effectiveness of existing liposomal carriers through their functionalization, allowed to propose a promising candidate for multifunctional nanoplatform based on liposomes and magnetic nanoparticles called magnetoliposomes. The presence of magnetic nanoparticles makes it possible to magnetically direct the liposomal carrier to the specific site, and appropriate magnetic field parameters can lead to controlled disintegration of the vesicle and release of the drug. The increasing variety of suggested platforms constantly provides new variants in the structure and mechanism of drug release, which enable the adjustment of the carrier's characteristics to the specific needs of cancer therapy.

Keywords: magnetoliposomes, drug delivery, controlled release, magnetic nanoparticles, magnetotherapy

1. Introduction

Cancer remains still a major problem worldwide, leading to many deaths. There are many available anticancer drugs that effectively work against tumors, but their dose in anticancer therapies is limited due to numerous side effects [1]. Currently, carriers known as drug delivery systems (DDS) are used to limit the administration of conventional drugs and improve the safety of pharmacological treatment of patients. According to the DDS definition, these are preparations that enable the controlled introduction and distribution of the drug in the organism [2]. The functionality and effectiveness of DDS consist of the stages related to the structure, that is, the

IntechOpen

synthesis enabling to obtain specific physicochemical properties of the carrier, the method of immobilizing the drug inside the structure, administration, delivery, and release of the content at a specific place and time [3].

Drug delivery systems allow for better use of anticancer compounds and greater control of the drug while it is circulating in the bloodstream, thereby significantly reducing drug's side effects on healthy tissues. The advantage of such systems over the original form of drugs improves bioavailability and systemic clearance by achieving the optimal concentration of the drug in the target tissue. Additionally, entrapment of drugs in the form of carriers may solve problems with their stability and solubility [4–6].

2. Drug delivery systems

Drug carriers are widely researched and used due to the wide variety of materials from which they can be proposed. Initially, the main challenge for DDS was to reduce the side effects of strong cytostatics that, in free form in the bloodstream, induced cytotoxic damage to healthy tissues, as well as in the target sites. Anthracyclines are the primary chemotherapy drugs used in breast cancer. Doxorubicin (DOX) is one example of an effective anticancer drug with adverse effects on many organs. The greatest clinical problem with the use of conventional anthracyclines is cardiovascular complications, which mainly concern patients with significant risk factors for the development of heart failure [7–9]. Pegylated liposomal doxorubicin under the name Doxil® is a commercially used form of an enclosed drug and was the first liposomal formulation approved by the US Food and Drug Administration (FDA) [10].

2.1 Liposomes

Due to their structure and pharmacokinetics, liposomes are widely used as carriers for anticancer drugs and are particularly advantageous due to the possibility of encapsulating both hydrophilic and hydrophobic drugs [11]. Selective action of liposomes within the tumor can be achieved by passive accumulation associated with the enhanced permeability and retention (EPR) effect [12, 13]. Their phospholipid structure also allows for the slow release of the active substance. Studies of liposomal doxorubicin indicate the lack of initial high peak plasma concentrations of doxorubicin, while the actual peak concentration of the cardiotoxic metabolite occurs later and is lower compared to the conventional form [14, 15]. The encapsulation of doxorubicin in liposomes makes it practically impossible to penetrate the wall of properly functioning capillaries in healthy tissues [16, 17]. Research confirms that drug encapsulation causes significantly fewer cardiovascular complications than the conventional form [18].

Nevertheless, with the current advancement of research, liposomal vesicles are insufficient as an independent carrier due to slow action, susceptibility to phagocytosis, and insufficient drug release at the tumor site. Significant efforts in designing and developing novel drug delivery systems for targeted cancer chemotherapy remain a significant challenge. The main direction is to improve the drug delivery system, which includes two main approaches. The first concerns active approach, which is targeted guidance of the drug carrier to the target site. The second is passive approach, in which passive accumulation of liposomes by the EPR

Name of product	Name of drug	Cancer type	Main composition	Refs
DaunoXome®	Daunorubicin	AIDS-related Kaposi's sarcoma	DSPC:Chol	[26]
Doxil®	Doxorubicin	Ovarian, breast, Kaposi's sarcoma	HSPC:Chol: MPEG-DSPE	[10, 27]
DepoCyt®	Cytarabine	Acute leukemia, meningeal lymphoma	DOPC:DPPG: Chol:triolein	[28]
Myocet®	Doxorubicin	Metastatic breast, ovarian, multiple myeloma, Kaposi's sarcoma	EPC:Chol	[15, 29]
Mepact®	Mifamurtide	Osteosarcoma, bone	DOPS:POPC	[30]
Marqibo®	Vincristine	Acute lymphoblastic leukemia	SM:Chol	[31, 32]
Lipoplatin™	Cisplatin	Pancreatic, lung	DPPG:PC: MPEG-DSPE: Chol	[33]
Onivyde™	Irinotecan	Pancreatic	DSPC:MPEG-DSPE:Chol	[34]
ThermoDox®	Doxorubicin	Liver, breast	DPPC:MSPC: MPEG-DSPE	[35]
Visudyne®	Verteporfin	Choroidal neovascularisation	EPG:DMPC	[36]

Abbreviations: distearoylphosphatidylcholine (DSPC); hydrogenated soy phosphatidylcholine (HSPC); methoxy polyethylene glycol (MPEG); distearoyl-sn-glycero-phosphoethanolamine (DSPE); dioleoylphosphatidylcholine (DOPC); dipalmitoylphosphatidylglycerol (DPPG); egg phosphatidylcholine (EPC); dioleoylphosphatidylserine (DOPS); palmitoyloleoylphosphatidylcholine (POPC); sphingomyelin (SM); phosphatidylcholine (PC); dipalmitoylphosphatidylcholine (DPPC); 1-myristoyl-2-stearoyl-sn-glycero-3-phosphocholine (MSPC); egg phosphatidylglycerol (EPG); dimyristoyl phosphatidylcholine (DMPC).

Table 1.
Summary of the commercial liposomal products.

effect is insufficient to ensure proper targeting due to imprecise and slow distribution. Moreover, not all tumors exhibit vascular porosity and a high degree of tumor vascularization [19–21]. Given the stability of the liposomal formulation, slow action prevents complete drug delivery and creates the need to optimize active targeting by functionalization with various targeting ligands, such as proteins, peptides, nucleic acids, or small molecules. The targeting strategy involving mainly ligand-coupled liposomes is based on obtaining tumor-specific targeting through the interaction between the ligand and the receptor overexpressed in cancer cells [22–25]. The potential of liposomes for such modifications has led to various patents, which are listed in **Table 1**.

A second approach to increase the efficiency of drug delivery using conventional liposomes is to induce a controlled release of the drug at a specific location and time using an internally or externally guided mechanism. The capsule disintegration mechanism is initiated by stimuli and is strictly dependent on the lipids building liposomal carriers. Thus, controlled leakage of drugs at the target site can be caused by specific external stimuli applied to specific liposomes sensitive to ultrasound, light, and temperature or by the use of specific biological features in tumor microenvironment such as low pH, enzymes, redox potential and hypoxia [37, 38].

3. Magnetoliposomes

In recent years, increasing attention has been paid to the application of an external magnetic field in directing the drug carriers to the target tissue with subsequent stimulated drug release from the carriers in this tissue. The great potential in this regard has led to the connection of liposomes with magnetic nanoparticles (MNP) forming nanostructures called magnetoliposomes (MLP). Their size ranges from 100 to 150 nm, but the final size depends on the method of liposome synthesis [39]. The potential applications of these relatively new carriers are increasingly recognized as providing significant biomedical possibilities both in the diagnosis and treatment of cancer and in monitoring the effectiveness of the therapy. The presence of magnetic nanoparticles enables magnetic targeting based on the selective guidance of the MLP to the target site and maintenance of the drug in the diseased tissue by applying a permanent magnet there. In addition, an alternating magnetic field (AMF) can be used as an exogenous stimulus to trigger a controlled drug release due to carrier degradation. Hereby, magnetoliposomes are an area of strong interest and research for the development and creation of new multifunctional magnetic nanomaterials with complex functions in drug delivery systems. This literature review is devoted to issues related to the types and methods of obtaining magnetoliposomes, and the next section is devoted to the advances and recent achievements in the field of controlled-release drug delivery with the use of magnetoliposomes [40, 41].

3.1 Types of magnetoliposomes

The magnetic properties of MLP allow magnetic targeting with a permanent magnet. For nanoparticles to meet specific properties and show a specific susceptibility to MF, it is important, however, that they have a strong magnetic moment randomly oriented at room temperature in the absence of the external magnetic field. This means using MNP, which are superparamagnetic, makes them prone to strong magnetization. When the magnetic field is applied, nanoparticles orient themselves towards the field but do not maintain permanent magnetization in the absence of MF. This behavior is due to the small size of nanoparticles, up to 10 nm, where these nanoparticles are single-domain with a single magnetic moment. In such a system, interactions between particles are weak, therefore, after removing the magnetic field, nanoparticles can return to the state of disorder. MNP also have other interesting features regarding their ability to modify the surface and create unique structures tailored to the variability of the magnetic field strength, which determines the specific mechanism of drug release from the carrier [42, 43].

Magnetic nanoparticles can be arranged differently in the structure of liposomes depending on the nature of their surface. Magnetoliposomes can be formed using three different approaches: encapsulation of hydrophilic nanoparticles in the aqueous core of liposomes, incorporation of hydrophobic nanoparticles into a phospholipid bilayer, and binding magnetic nanoparticles to the surface of liposomes (**Figure 1**). The above-mentioned designs should be selected according to the application, as each has its own advantages and disadvantages. For example, the presence of both nanoparticles and drug inside liposomes reduces the drug loading capacity of such carriers. However, this is the most well-known method due to the ease of incorporation of nanoparticles. In turn, the deposition of nanoparticles in the membrane poses some limitations concerning the capacity and size of the bilayer. Its thickness varies

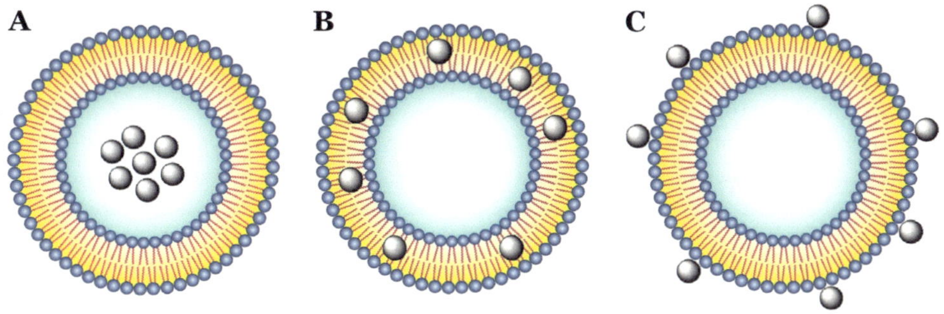

Figure 1.
Schematic representation of the main types of magnetoliposome structure related to the distribution of magnetic nanoparticles: encapsulation of hydrophilic nanoparticles in the aqueous core of the liposomes (A); incorporation of hydrophobic nanoparticles in the phospholipid bilayer (B); and bonding of magnetic nanoparticles on the surface of liposomes (C).

around 6 nm, so only suitably small and well-separated nanoparticles are introduced. Under the influence of the presence of nanoparticles, the bilayer convexes and becomes stiffer. Regardless of the point of introduction, it is necessary to coat the nanoparticles to prevent their aggregation and to improve the efficiency of incorporation into liposomes. MNP are most often coated with citric acid as hydrophilic introduced inside liposomes or with oleic acid, oleylamine as hydrophobic in the phospholipid bilayer [44, 45].

3.2 Methods of magnetoliposomes preparation

The preparation of magnetoliposomes is divided into two separate steps, involving the initial synthesis of magnetic nanoparticles and the subsequent combination with lipids in the proper synthesis of magnetoliposomes [46].

3.2.1 Synthesis of magnetic nanoparticles

The methods of producing nanoparticles can be divided into bottom-up methods, consisting in building a nanometric structure from individual atoms or molecules, and top-down methods, consisting in grinding a micrometric structure to the nanometric scale. To obtain metal nanoparticles with high stability and high chemical purity, as well as of the desired sizes, bottom-up methods are used, including chemical strategies, such as co-precipitation, thermal decomposition, sol–gel, hydrothermal and solvothermal methods, and the synthesis of microemulsions [47, 48]. Co-precipitation is the most common method because it is characterized by simplicity, high efficiency, and low cost. Undoubtedly, its advantage is also the possibility of producing nanoparticles of different chemical compositions and controlling the size of the obtained nanoparticles, which determines the achievement of the desired superparamagnetic properties. The morphology of nanoparticles and their stability can be controlled by selecting appropriate synthesis parameters, such as metal salt concentration, stabilizer concentration, and the molar ratio of the reducer and metal salt. For example, by increasing the molar ratio of salt to the reductant, it is possible to create many nuclei and, as a result, to obtain small, monodisperse nanoparticles [49].

Iron oxide-based nanoparticles are a class of great biomedical importance due to their good magnetic properties, stability, biocompatibility, and the possibility of chemical modification [50]. These nanoparticles are most often obtained by the aforementioned co-precipitation method, which consists of the co-precipitation of a stoichiometric mixture of iron and ferrous salts in an aqueous medium and the absence of oxygen. Carefully planned synthesis procedures (water-phase co-precipitation and thermal decomposition from organic precursors) will yield iron-based magnetic nanoparticles with controlled sizes and surface properties suitable for later use as a "vector" to guide drug-loaded magnetoliposomes in an external magnetic field and initiate drug release in an alternating magnetic field [51]. For example, various ferrite nanoparticles were synthesized by co-precipitation, including ferrites doped with manganese, calcium, magnesium, and nickel [52]. The previously prepared magnetic nanoparticles are supplied with lipids during liposome synthesis and, depending on the surface nature, hydrophilic or hydrophobic, are incorporated into the interior or bilayers of magnetoliposomes, respectively [53].

3.2.2 Synthesis of liposomes and magnetic liposomes

Magnetoliposomes are created during the synthesis of liposomes, which are modified with magnetic nanoparticles by administering them together with a lipid mixture. The choice of the method of liposome preparation depends on the method of using the obtained vesicles. The simplest and most used technique is the hydration of a thin lipid/nanoparticle film. In this process, lipids and MNP are first dissolved in a volatile organic solvent and a thin layer is formed at the bottom of the container after the solvent is evaporated under nitrogen. The sample is then rehydrated with a phosphate buffer. Using this method, a heterogeneous suspension of multilayer magnetoliposomes with a diameter of 0.1 μm to 10 μm is obtained. However, the main disadvantage of this synthesis is the low encapsulation efficiency of hydrophilic drugs (5–20%) [54, 55]. Next method of magnetic liposome preparation includes, among others, evaporation using the reverse phase technique, in which a mixture consisting of two phases: lipids and nanoparticles are dissolved in an organic solvent and a buffer is subjected to short sonication. The solvent is then removed under low pressure to form a sticky gel. The final step of the procedure, involving the removal of residual solvent on a rotary evaporator under reduced pressure, produces bubbles with a large size distribution. They are characterized by a high encapsulation efficiency of up to 65% in a solution with low ionic strength. The disadvantage of the method, however, is that the entrapped drug dissolved in the buffer contacts the organic phase. Additionally, intensive sonication may damage the structure of the closed substance [56]. Another method of magnetoliposomes preparation is the rapid injection of lipids with magnetic nanoparticles dissolved in ethanol into the aqueous solution. This procedure results in a heterogeneous suspension of vesicles with a diameter of 30 to 110 nm. The obtained magnetic liposome suspension is diluted and may contain traces of ethanol [55, 57]. In turn, the freeze-thaw technique allows one to obtain small single-layer magnetoliposomes. After sonication, they are quickly frozen in liquid nitrogen and slowly thawed in water, as a result of this process liposomes fuse and are characterized by a loading efficiency of 20–30% [57]. Similar to the ethanol injection described above, an ether solution or ether/methanol solution of lipids and MNP can be slowly injected into the buffer at elevated temperature under reduced pressure. A heterogeneous suspension of magnetoliposomes with a diameter of 70 to 190 nm is formed. As with the reverse phase evaporation technique, the enclosed drug is exposed to phase mixing with an organic solvent at high temperatures [56, 57]. Some of the above MLP preparation techniques result in multilayer and single-layer vesicles with a large size distribution. Due to the efficient permeability of small carriers to tumor cells, homogeneous vesicles in the range of 100–200 nm are preferred. In order to homogenize the obtained heterogeneous mixture, MLP extrusion through polycarbonate membrane filters with a defined pore diameter is used. As a result, the obtained phospholipid vesicles are characterized by a small size distribution. Additionally, this method is fast, cheap, and allows obtaining even small, unilamellar liposomes of 100 nm in size. The breaking down of the vesicles into smaller structures can also be obtained by the action of ultrasound, which can complement the above techniques to increase the effectiveness of MLP preparation [55].

The discussed methods assume the closure of compounds during the synthesis of magnetoliposomes. In this case, we can talk about the so-called passive loading. However, some compounds have ionizable groups that exhibit hydrophobic and hydrophilic properties depending on the pH of the solution and may not be efficiently encapsulated in liposomes due to their diffusion through the phospholipid membrane. In such a case, they can be encapsulated in liposomes with high efficiency, even above 90%, after the formation of the liposomes using the active loading technique. In this method, liposomes are prepared with their internal pH suitable for ionizing the drug, which in this non-ionized form can passively diffuse through the lipid membrane from the external solution into the liposomes. As a result, the drug after penetration into the liposome becomes ionized and is no longer able to re-diffuse through the phospholipid bilayer [58, 59].

3.3 Mechanisms of drug release from magnetoliposomes

So far, in the chapter, we discussed the methodology of magnetoliposomes and their modification to obtain an effective magnetic field-assisted drug delivery system. In addition to the selective action of the constant magnetic field, enabling the efficient accumulation of carriers within the tumor tissue, it is possible to obtain, on-demand, the release of drugs enclosed in the carriers. Then, an alternating magnetic field is used which, by changing the behavior of nanoparticles, initiates the degradation of the carrier and the outflow of the drug. The susceptibility of nanoparticles to AMF results from their superparamagnetic behavior, for which the physicochemical properties of these nanomaterials and strict control of parameters during synthesis are responsible. Only superparamagnetic nanoparticles are capable of efficient, local release of the drug from the carriers. How the degradation of the magnetoliposomes takes place depends on the parameters of the magnetic field, where special attention is focused on the use of low or high frequency [60].

3.3.1 Magnetic hyperthermia

In magnetic hyperthermia, the exposure of magnetic nanoparticles to the magnetic field will result in their magnetization, and the supplied amount of magnetic field energy will be converted into heat. In the case of single-domain, superparamagnetic iron oxide nanoparticles (SPION), relaxation losses related to the rotation of the magnetic moment inside the nanoparticle (Nelson) and a lesser extent to the physical rotation of the entire nanoparticle (Brown) may cause local heating of the magnetoliposomes. Taking into account the short relaxation time, an alternating high-frequency magnetic field (AMF-HF), 50–400 kHz, is used [61]. In this case, the heat released under the influence of nanoparticles placed in a magnetic field is a factor that initiates the degradation of the liposomal carrier. Liposomes are characterized by a phase transition temperature that keeps the drug inside the structure. When these liposomes are loaded with magnetic nanoparticles and drugs, an interesting drug delivery system can be created. The energy supplied from the magnetic system in the form of heat, after exceeding the threshold value Tm, causes a phase transition in the phospholipid bilayer. This magnetocaloric effect enables the activation of drug release from MLP in the presence of AMF by locally increasing the temperature in the membrane and inducing changes in liposome permeability, which changes with increasing temperature. Under these conditions, the order of phospholipid molecules changes, which results in destabilization and an increase in the fluidity of the membrane. Leaks, that appear as a result of such changes, allow dissolved drugs to pass through the membrane. The packing of lipids depends on the degree of saturation of fatty acid residues and the number of carbon atoms that build them, which translates into different Tm values of individual lipids. Therefore, when designing carriers, thermosensitive lipids are selected that are able to release the drug even with a slight increase in temperature. Magnetic nanoparticles can be used to generate both mild hyperthermia (42–46°C) and high-temperature hyperthermia (> 46°C). However, even under milder conditions of temperature increase, neoplastic tissues are exposed to it, because they are more sensitive to higher temperatures than normal cells, and as a result, local hypoxia and acidification of the tumor occur, and eventually apoptosis. Higher temperature hyperthermia causes immediate tissue necrosis through dehydration, protein denaturation, and damage to cell membranes (thermal ablation) and is rarely used due to its negative impact on the viability of healthy cells. The undoubted advantage of using magnetic hyperthermia among magnetoliposomes is the possibility of inducing heat only in a strictly defined volume, in which magnetic nanoparticles are located. However, it should be noted that a living organism cannot be exposed to an alternating magnetic field of any high-intensity H and frequency f, because eddy currents can be induced in it, leading to heating of the whole body or a significant part of it. Therefore, in treatments with the use of AMF, these values are strictly limited to the safe range, in accordance with the Brezovich criterion, which requires $H{\cdot}f < 4.85 \times 10^{8}\ Am^{-1}\,s^{-1}$ [62–64].

3.3.2 Mechanical degradation

An alternative, relatively new approach to activating drug release from magnetoliposomes in the presence of AMF is the degradation of the carrier by mechanical means. This manner of controlled drug release is effected by using a low-frequency alternating magnetic field (AMF-LF). Under the influence of a low-frequency < 50 Hz, the movements of the superparamagnetic magnetic nanoparticles become dominant, which leads to the mechanical disruption of the lipid bilayer of the vesicles and the release of the drug from the liposomes. Currently, there is growing interest in research on the controlled release of a drug from magnetic carriers under the influence of AMF-LF. The disintegration process takes place without sudden increases in temperature and without magnetically induced eddy currents, preventing damage and reducing the viability of healthy cells surrounding the tumor. A significant advantage of this mechanism over magnetic hyperthermia is also a significant reduction in the parameters of the magnetic field, which in this case are within the acceptable ranges of conventional magnetotherapy, and therefore can be considered a safe dose [37, 65].

The above reasons prompted us to develop a selective delivery of doxorubicin to cancer cells supported by a low-frequency magnetic field with the use of magnetoliposomes as drug carriers [66]. To the best of our knowledge, the magnetoliposome design we propose has been optimized and adapted to a specific application. Moreover, the physicochemical characteristics of the carrier met the criteria for drug delivery systems, which are discussed in more detail in our article. The main research object was the use of magnetomechanical activation for controlled drug release, which we reported for the first time in 2016 by Joniec et al., see [67]. For further purposes and biological studies, degradation of the carrier under unheated conditions was desirable to avoid synergistic cytotoxic effects caused by released doxorubicin and elevated temperature. The selection of lipids took into account the possibility of obtaining MLP with appropriate physicochemical properties and good stability in the conditions of cell culture, as well as different conditions in the tumor environment. We used passive loading of the drug into the aqueous phase of the liposome, which compared to active loading has a lower efficiency of drug encapsulation. Thus, in order to increase this final efficiency, we synthesized hydrophobic SPION. As a result, during the incorporation into liposomes, they locate in the hydrophobic phospholipid bilayer, leaving a free internal space for the drug. Moreover, such separation may prevent interaction between the vibrating SPION and the drug. For loaded to the interior of the liposome bilayer, their magnetic movement, limited only to the membrane, may facilitate the degradation of the carrier and thus increase the drug release efficiency. We have successfully tested the *in vitro* effect of magnetoliposomes loaded with doxorubicin as a potent cytostatic drug, on a cancerous human breast cell line. The obtained nanocarriers were susceptible to an alternating magnetic field in low frequency, released a significant amount of drug, and caused a highly efficient reduction in the viability of cancerous cells in comparison to control without exposure to this magnetic field (**Figure 2**).

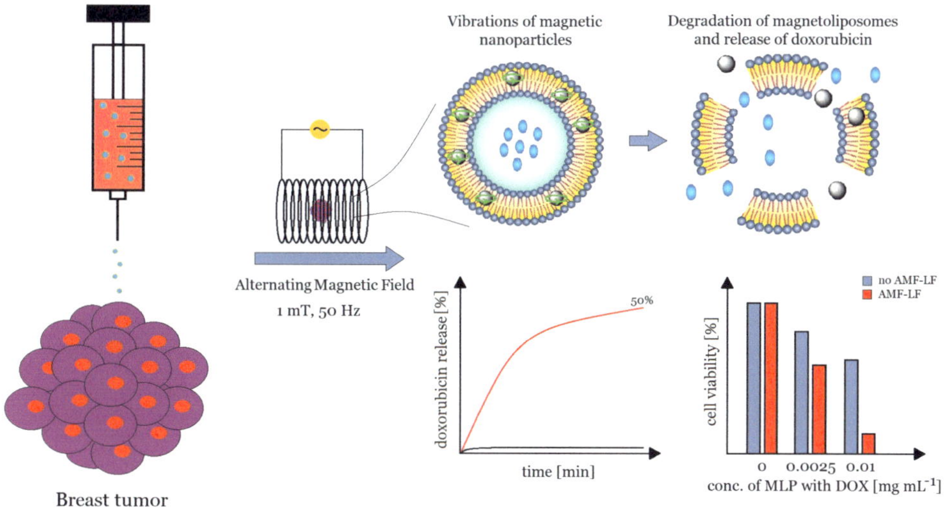

Figure 2.
Schematic illustration showing the research concept of magnetoliposomes as magnetically assisted drug nanocarriers.

4. Advances in anticancer drug delivery system using magnetoliposomes

In recent years, the worldwide progress in research has been significant and has led to new advances in the field of controlled-release drug delivery using magnetoliposomes. Modifications in the design of carrier structures tended to create multifunctional platforms to improve parameters, including drug maintenance, target accumulation, and active drug release mechanism. Several innovative solutions from the last 3 years are presented below.

The research presented in the article by Cintra et al. in 2022, see [68] demonstrates the antitumor properties of magnetoliposomes that have been functionalized with a selective ligand to actively target the tumor. Folic acid was used to modify the surface of magnetoliposomes. The potential effect of drug accumulation into neoplastic cells is related to the overexpression of folic acid receptors by some neoplasms, including ovarian cancer [69]. The release of the drug from MLP took place with the participation of heat released by an alternating magnetic field under magnetic hyperthermia.

Another example of the use of magnetoliposomes and magnetic hyperthermia was the study by Riberio et al. in 2020, see [70]. In this example, an interesting approach was the multi-drug loading into magnetoliposomes. Magnetic nanoparticles, gemcitabine, and paclitaxel were encapsulated in thermosensitive liposomes with high efficiency and showed equally efficient drug release from preparations exposed to AMF-HF. In addition, the separated and combined cytotoxic effects of loaded magnetoliposomes and magnetic hyperthermia on breast cancer cells were investigated. Based on the presented work, the authors stated that drug-loaded magnetoliposomes may have the potential for combination therapy, including hyperthermia and controlled release of chemotherapeutic drugs.

The development of stimulus-sensitive DDS is a current area of cancer therapy research by Riberio et al., see [71]. The authors have developed magnetic liposomes adequate for temperature and pH-triggered anticancer drug release in the tumor environment in conjunction with magnetic hyperthermia. Two new anticancer thienopyridine derivatives have been successfully enclosed in magnetoliposomes and the results have confirmed the efficiency of drug delivery by loaded nanocarriers under various pH and temperature conditions.

Departing from the use of AMF-HF and magnetic hyperthermia to release encapsulated compounds on demand, Trilli et al., see [72] proposed magnetoliposomes sensitive to low-intensity magnetic fields. The use of low-intensity pulsed electromagnetic fields (PEMF) provided magnetomechanical activation and efficient content release. In particular, the authors devoted attention to investigating the effect of bilayer packing on the ability of MLP with oleic acid-coated MNP enclosed in a bilayer to respond to PEMF application. For this purpose, magnetoliposomes with different lipid composition and the degree of order of the phospholipid bilayer were compared. The effectiveness of the magnetic triggering was greatest with highly ordered bilayers that are unable to suppress the disturbance caused by MNP movement.

5. Conclusion

In summary, the growing variety of proposed platforms constantly provides new variants in the structure and mechanism of drug release, which enable the adaptation of the carrier to the specific needs of the therapy. The number of literature reports on the development of new multifunctional drug carriers is constantly growing.

However, due to the development of more precise anticancer therapies, increasingly advanced solutions are being sought. Nanotechnology can offer many opportunities, progress in this field is constantly developing methods of producing and studying magnetoliposomes.

Acknowledgements

This work was implemented as a part of Operational Project Knowledge Education Development 2014–2020 cofinanced by the European Social Fund.

This work has been supported by Warsaw University of Technology and University of Warsaw.

Conflict of interest

The authors declare no conflict of interest.

Author details

Edyta Maroń[1,2], Paweł Krysiński[2] and Michał Chudy[1*]

1 Faculty of Chemistry, Warsaw University of Technology, Chair of Medical Biotechnology, Warsaw, Poland

2 Faculty of Chemistry, University of Warsaw, Laboratory of Electrochemistry, Warsaw, Poland

*Address all correspondence to: chudziak@ch.pw.edu.pl

References

[1] Bargahi N, Ghasemali S, Jahandar-Lashaki S, Nazari A. Recent advances for cancer detection and treatment by microfluidic technology, review and update. Biol. Proced. Online. 2022;**24**(1):5. DOI: 10.1186/s12575-022-00166-y

[2] Jain KK. An overview of drug delivery systems. In: Jain KK, editor. Drug Delivery Systems. Method Mol. Biol. New York: Humana; 2020. p. 2059. DOI: 10.1007/978-1-4939-9798-5_1

[3] Boverhof DR, Bramante CM, Butala JH, Clancy SF, Lafranconi M, West J, et al. Comparative assessment of na-nomaterial definitions and safety evaluation considerations. Regulatory Toxicology and Pharmacology. 2015;**73**:137-150. DOI: 10.1016/j.yrtph.2015.06.001

[4] Lavik EB, Kuppermann BD, Humayun MS. Drug delivery. In: Hinton DR, editor. Basic Science and Translation to Therapy. United States: W.B. Saunders; 2013. pp. 734-745. DOI: 10.1016/B978-1-4557-0737-9.00038-2

[5] Garg NK, Tandel N, Jadon RS, Tyagi RK, Katare OP. Lipid-polymer hybrid nanocarrier-mediated cancer therapeutics: Current status and future directions. Drug Discovery Today. 2018;**23**(9):1610-1621. DOI: 10.1016/j.drudis.2018.05.033

[6] Sohail M, Guo W, Li Z, Xu H, Zhao F, Chen D, et al. Nanocarrier-based drug delivery system for cancer therapeutics: A review of the last decade. Current Medicinal Chemistry. 2021;**28**(19):3753-3772. DOI: 10.2174/0929867327666201005111722

[7] Tacar O, Sriamornsak P, Dass CR. Doxorubicin: An update on anticancer molecular action, toxicity and novel drug delivery systems. The Journal of Pharmacy and Pharmacology. 2013;**65**(2):157-170. DOI: 10.1111/j.2042-7158.2012.01567.x

[8] Malato A, Saccullo G, Fazio G, Vergara B, Raso S, Guarneri GP, et al. Drug-related cardiotoxicity for the treatment of haematological malignancies in elderly. Current Pharmaceutical Design. 2010;**16**(26):2872-2879. DOI: 10.2174/138161210793176446

[9] Trucillo P. Drug carriers: Classification, administration, release profiles, and industrial approach. PRO. 2021;**9**:470. DOI: 10.3390/pr9030470

[10] Porche DJ. Liposomal doxorubicin (Doxil). The Journal of the Association of Nurses in AIDS Care. 1996;**7**(2):55-59. DOI: 10.1016/S1055-3290(96)80016-1

[11] Abu Lila AS, Ishida T. Liposomal delivery systems: Design optimization and current applications. Biological & Pharmaceutical Bulletin. 2017;**40**(1):1-10. DOI: 10.1248/bpb.b16-00624

[12] Danhier F. To exploit the tumor microenvironment: Since the EPR effect fails in the clinic, what is the future of nanomedicine? Journal of Controlled Release. 2016;**28**(244):108-121. DOI: 10.1016/j.jconrel.2016.11.015

[13] Maeda H, Wu J, Sawa T, Matsumura Y, Hori K. Tumor vascular permeability and the EPR effect in macromolecular therapeutics: A review. Journal of Controlled Release. 2000;**65**(1-2):271-284. DOI: 10.1016/s0168-3659(99)00248-5

[14] Mayer LD, Tai LC, Bally MB, Mitilenes GN, Ginsberg RS, Cullis PR.

Characterization of liposomal systems containing doxorubicin entrapped in response to pH gradients. Biochimica et Biophysica Acta. 1990;**1025**:143-151. DOI: 10.1016/0005-2736(90)90091-2

[15] Marty M. Liposomal doxorubicin (Myocet™) and conventional anthracyclines: A comparison. The Breast. 2001;**10**:28-33. DOI: 10.1016/S0960-9776(01)80005-9

[16] Tardi PG, Boman NL, Cullis PR. Liposomal doxorubicin. Journal of Drug Targeting. 1996;**4**(3):129-140. DOI: 10.3109/10611869609015970

[17] Makwana V, Karanjia J, Haselhorst T, Anoopkumar-Dukie S, Rudrawar S. Liposomal doxorubicin as targeted delivery platform: Current trends in surface functionalization. International Journal of Pharmaceutics. 2021;**25**(593):120117. DOI: 10.1016/j.ijpharm.2020.120117

[18] Batist G, Harris L, Azarnia N, Lee LW, Daza-Ramirez P. Improved anti-tumor response rate with decreased cardiotoxicity of non-pegylated liposomal doxorubicin compared with conventional doxorubicin in first-line treatment of metastatic breast cancer in patients who had received prior adjuvant doxorubicin: Results of a retrospective analysis. Anti-Cancer Drugs. 2006;**17**(5):587-595. DOI:10.1097/00001813-200606000-00014

[19] Qamar Z, Qizilbash FF, Iqubal MK, Ali A, Narang JK, Ali J, et al. Nano-based drug delivery system: Recent strategies for the treatment of ocular disease and future perspective. Recent Patents on Drug Delivery & Formulation. 2019;**13**(4):246-254. DOI: 10.2174/1872211314666191224115211

[20] Meng W, He C, Hao Y, Wang L, Li L, Zhu G. Prospects and challenges of extracellular vesicle-based drug delivery system: Considering cell source. Drug Delivery. 2020;**27**(1):585-598. DOI: 10.1080/10717544.2020.1748758

[21] Heidarli E, Dadashzadeh S, Haeri A. State of the art of stimuli-responsive liposomes for cancer therapy. Iran. J. Pharm. Res. 2017;**16**(4):1273-1304. DOI: PMCID: PMC5843293

[22] Mertz D, Sandre O, Bégin-Colin S. Drug releasing nanoplatforms activated by alternating magnetic fields. Biochimica et Biophysica Acta - General Subjects. 2017;**1861**(6):1617-1641. DOI: 10.1016/j.bbagen.2017.02.025

[23] Yang B, Song BP, Shankar S, Guller A, Deng W. Recent advances in liposome formulations for breast cancer therapeutics. Cellular and Molecular Life Sciences. 2021;**78**(13):5225-5243. DOI: 10.1007/s00018-021-03850-6

[24] Veloso SRS, Andrade RGD, Castanheira EMS. Magnetoliposomes: Recent advances in the field of controlled drug delivery. Expert Opinion on Drug Delivery. 2021;**18**(10):1323-1334. DOI: 10.1080/17425247.2021.1915983

[25] Rajabi M, Mousa SA. Lipid nanoparticles and their application in Nanomedicine. Current Pharmaceutical Biotechnology. 2016;**17**(8):662-672. DOI: 10.2174/1389201017666160415155457

[26] Offidani M, Corvatta L, Centurioni R, Leoni F, Malerba L, Mele A, et al. High-dose daunorubicin as liposomal compound (Daunoxome) in elderly patients with acute lymphoblastic leukemia. The Hematology Journal. 2003;**4**(1):47-53. DOI: 10.1038/sj.thj.6200222

[27] Barenholz Y. Doxil® — The first FDA-approved nano-drug: Lessons learned. Journal of Controlled Release. 2012;**160**(2):117-134. DOI: 10.1016/j.jconrel.2012.03.020

[28] Murry DJ, Blaney SM. Clinical pharmacology of encapsulated sustained-release cytarabine. The Annals of Pharmacotherapy. 2000;**34**(10):1173-1178. DOI: 10.1345/aph.19347

[29] Balazsovits JA, Mayer LD, Bally MB, Cullis PR, McDonell M, Ginsberg RS, et al. Analysis of the effect of liposome encapsulation on the vesicant properties, acute and cardiac toxicities, and antitumor efficacy of doxorubicin. Cancer Chemotherapy and Pharmacology. 1989;**23**(2):81-86. DOI: 10.1007/BF00273522

[30] Vail DM, MacEwen EG, Kurzman ID, Dubielzig RR, Helfand SC, Kisseberth WC, et al. Liposome-encapsulated muramyl tripeptide phosphatidylethanolamine adjuvant immunotherapy for splenic hemangiosarcoma in the dog: A randomized multi-institutional clinical trial. Clinical Cancer Research. 1995;**1**(10):1165-1170

[31] Silverman JA, Deitcher SR. Marqibo® (vincristine sulfate liposome injection) improves the pharmacokinetics and pharmacodynamics of vincristine. Cancer Chemotherapy and Pharmacology. 2013;**71**(3):555-564. DOI: 10.1007/s00280-012-2042-4

[32] Johnston MJ, Semple SC, Klimuk SK, Edwards K, Eisenhardt ML, Leng EC, et al. Therapeutically optimized rates of drug release can be achieved by varying the drug-to-lipid ratio in liposomal vincristine formulations. Biochimica et Biophysica Acta. 2006;**1758**(1):55-64. DOI: 10.1016/j.bbamem.2006.01.009

[33] Stathopoulos GP, Boulikas T, Vougiouka M, Deliconstantinos G, Rigatos S, Darli E, et al. Pharmacokinetics and adverse reactions of a new liposomal cisplatin (Lipoplatin): Phase I study. Oncology Reports. 2005;**13**(4):589-595

[34] Bulbake U, Doppalapudi S, Kommineni N, Khan W. Liposomal formulations in clinical use: An updated review. Pharmaceutics. 2017;**9**(2):12. DOI: 10.3390/pharmaceutics9020012

[35] Chen J, He CQ, Lin AH, Gu W, Chen ZP, Li W, et al. Thermosensitive liposomes with higher phase transition temperature for targeted drug delivery to tumor. International Journal of Pharmaceutics. 2014;**475**(1-2):408-415. DOI: 10.1016/j.ijpharm.2014.09.009

[36] Saraf S, Jain A, Tiwari A, Verma A, Panda PK, Jain SK. Advances in liposomal drug delivery to cancer: An overview. J. Drug Deliv. Sci. Technol. 2020;**56**:101549. DOI: 10.1016/j.jddst.2020.101549

[37] Nappini S, Bonini M, Bombelli FB, Pineider F, Sangregorio C, Baglioni P, et al. Controlled drug release under a low frequency magnetic field: Effect of the citrate coating on magnetoliposomes stability. Soft Matter. 2011;7:1025-1037. DOI: 10.1039/C0SM00789G

[38] Guo H, Chen W, Sun X, Liu YN, Li J, Wang J. Theranostic magnetoliposomes coated by carboxymethyl dextran with controlled release by low-frequency alternating magnetic field. Carbohydrate Polymers. 2015;**118**:209-217. DOI: 10.1016/j.carbpol.2014.10.076

[39] Bakandritsos A, Fatourou AG, Fatouros DG. Magnetoliposomes and their potential in the intelligent drug-delivery field. Therapeutic Delivery. 2012;**3**(12):1469-1482. DOI: 10.4155/tde.12.129

[40] Nappini S, Fogli S, Castroflorio B, Bonini M, Baldelli Bombelli F, Baglioni P. Magnetic field responsive drug release from magnetoliposomes in biological fluids. Journal of Materials Chemistry B. 2016;**4**(4):716-725. DOI: 10.1039/c5tb02191j

[41] Rodrigues ARO, Almeida BG, Rodrigues JM, Queiroz MJRP, Calhelha RC, Ferreira ICFR, et al. Magnetoliposomes as carriers for promising antitumor thieno[3,2-b]pyridin-7-arylamines: Photophysical and biological studies. RSC Advances. 2017;7:15352-15361. DOI: 10.1039/C7RA00447H

[42] Tomitaka A, Takemura Y, Huang Z, Roy U, Nair M. Magnetoliposomes in controlled-release drug delivery systems. Critical Reviews in Biomedical Engineering. 2019;**47**(6):495-505. DOI: 10.1615/CritRevBiomedEng.2020033002

[43] Wahajuddin AS. Superparamagnetic iron oxide nanoparticles: Magnetic nanoplatforms as drug carriers. International Journal of Nanomedicine. 2012;7:3445-3471. DOI: 10.2147/IJN.S30320

[44] Monnier CA, Burnand D, Rothen-Rutishauser B, Lattuada M, Petri-Fink A. Magnetoliposomes: Opportunities and challenges. Eur. J. Nanomed. 2014;**6**:201-215. DOI: 10.1515/ejnm-2014-0042

[45] Soenen SJ, Velde GV, Ketkar-Atre A, Himmelreich U, De Cuyper M. Magnetoliposomes as magnetic resonance imaging contrast agents. Wires. Nanomed. Nanobi. 2011;**3**(2):197-211. DOI: 10.1002/wnan.122

[46] Faria MR, Cruz MM, Gonçalves MC, Carvalho A, Feio G, Martins MB. Synthesis and characterization of magnetoliposomes for MRI contrast enhancement. International Journal of Pharmaceutics. 2013;**446**(1-2):183-190. DOI: 10.1016/j.ijpharm.2013.02.025

[47] Majidi S, Sehrig FZ, Farkhani SM, Goloujeh MS, Akbarzadeh A. Current methods for synthesis of magnetic nanoparticles. Artif. Cells Nanomed. Biotechnol. 2016;**44**(2):722-734. DOI: 10.3109/21691401.2014.982802

[48] Ramimoghadam D, Bagheri S, Hamid SBA. Progress in electrochemical synthesis of magnetic iron oxide nanoparticles. Journal of Magnetism and Magnetic Materials. 2014;**368**:207-229. DOI: 10.1016/j.jmmm.2014.05.015

[49] Babooram K. Novel solution routes to ferroelectrics and relaxors. In: Ye Z-G, editor. Handbook of Advanced Dielectric, Piezoelectric and Ferroelectric Materials. Materials Science. Cambridge, England: Woodhead Publishing; 2008. p. 852. DOI: 10.1533/9781845694005.7.852

[50] Lattuada M, Hatton TA. Functionalization of monodisperse magnetic nanoparticles. Langmuir. 2007;**23**(4):2158-2168. DOI: 10.1021/la062092x

[51] Mahdavi M, Ahmad MB, Haron MJ, Namvar F, Nadi B, Rahman MZ, et al. Synthesis, surface modification and characterisation of biocompatible magnetic iron oxide nanoparticles for biomedical applications. Molecules. 2013;**18**(7):7533-7548. DOI: 10.3390/molecules18077533

[52] Cardoso BD, Rio ISR, Rodrigues ARO, et al. Magnetoliposomes containing magnesium ferrite nanoparticles as nanocarriers for the model drug curcumin. Royal Society Open Science. 2018;**5**(10):181017. DOI: 10.1098/rsos.181017

[53] Amstad E, Gillich T, Bilecka I, Textor M, Reimhult E. Ultrastable iron oxide nanoparticle colloidal suspensions using dispersants with catechol-derived anchor groups. Nano Letters. 2009;**9**(12):4042-4048. DOI: 10.1021/nl902212q

[54] Shashi K, Satinder K, Bharat P. A complete review on: Liposomes. Int. Res. J. Pharm. 2012;**3**:10-16. DOI: 10.46956/ijihd.vi.116

[55] Vishvakrama P, Sharma S. Liposomes: An overview. J. Drug Deliv. Ther. 2014;**4**:47-55. DOI: 10.22270/jddt.v0i0.843

[56] Dua JS, Rana AC, Bhandari AK. Liposome: Methods of preparation and applications. Int. J. Pharm. Stud. Res. 2012;**3**:14-20

[57] Allen TM, Cullis PR. Liposomal drug delivery systems: From concept to clinical applications. Advanced Drug Delivery Reviews. 2013;**65**(1):36-48. DOI: 10.1016/j.addr.2012.09.037

[58] Gubernator J. Active methods of drug loading into liposomes: Recent strategies for stable drug entrapment and increased in vivo activity. Expert Opinion on Drug Delivery. 2011;**8**(5):565-580. DOI: 10.1517/17425247.2011.566552

[59] Sharma A, Sharma US. Liposomes in drug delivery: Progress and limitations. International Journal of Pharmaceutics. 1997;**54**(2):123-140. DOI: 10.1016/S0378-5173(97)00135-X

[60] McNeil SE. Nanoparticle therapeutics: A personal perspective. Wires. Nanomed. Nanobi. 2009;**1**(3):264-271. DOI: 10.1002/wnan.6

[61] Rosensweig RE. Heating magnetic fluid with alternating magnetic field. Journal of Magnetism and Magnetic Materials. 2002;**252**:370-374. DOI: 10.1016/S0304-8853(02)00706-0

[62] Robinson R, Gerlach W, Ghandehari H. Comparative effect of gold nanorods and nanocages for prostate tumor hyperthermia. Journal of Controlled Release. 2015;**220**:245-252. DOI: 10.1016/j.jconrel.2015.10.036

[63] Guo Y, Zhang Y, Ma J, Li Q, Li Y, Zhou X, et al. Light/magnetic hyperthermia triggered drug released from multi-functional thermo-sensitive magnetoliposomes for precise cancer synergetic theranostics. Journal of Controlled Release. 2018;**28**(272):145-158. DOI: 10.1016/j.jconrel.2017.04.028

[64] Rodrigues ARO, Ramos JMF, Gomes IT, Almeida BG, Araújo JP, Queiroz M-JRP, et al. Magnetoliposomes based on manganese ferrite nanoparticles as nanocarriers for antitumor drugs. RSC Advances. 2016;**6**:17302-17313. DOI: 10.1039/C5RA27058H

[65] Nappini S, Al Kayal T, Berti D, Norden B, Baglioni P. Magnetically triggered release from Giant Unilamellar vesicles: Visualization by means of confocal microscopy. Journal of Physical Chemistry Letters. 2011;**2**:713-718. DOI: 10.1021/jz2000936

[66] Szuplewska A, Rękorajska A, Pocztańska E, Krysiński P, Dybko A, Chudy M. Magnetic field-assisted selective delivery of doxorubicin to cancer cells using magnetoliposomes as drug nanocarriers. Nanotechnology. 2019;**30**:315101. DOI: 10.1088/1361-6528/ab19d3

[67] Joniec A, Sek S, Krysinski P. Magnetoliposomes as potential carriers of doxorubicin to Tumours. Chemistry. 2016;**22**(49):17715-17724. DOI: 10.1002/chem.201602809

[68] Cintra ER, Hayasaki TG, Sousa-Junior AA, Silva ACG, Valadares MC, Bakuzis AF, et al. Folate-targeted PEGylated Magnetoliposomes for hyperthermia-mediated controlled release of doxorubicin. Frontiers

in Pharmacology. 2022;**13**:854430. DOI: 10.3389/fphar.2022.854430

[69] Kukowska-Latallo JF, Candido KA, Cao Z, Nigavekar SS, Majoros IJ, Thomas TP, et al. Nanoparticle targeting of anticancer drug improves therapeutic response in animal model of human epithelial cancer. Cancer Research. 2005;**65**:5317-5324. DOI: 10.1158/0008-5472.CAN-04-3921

[70] Ribeiro RFL, Ferreira RV, Pedersoli DC, Paiva PRP, Cunha PS, Goes AM, et al. Cytotoxic effect of thermosensitive magnetoliposomes loaded with gemcitabine and paclitaxel on human primary breast cancer cells (MGSO-3 line). Journal of Nanoparticle Research. 2020;**22**:172. DOI: 10.1007/s11051-020-04833-7

[71] Ribeiro BC, Alvarez CAR, Alves BC, Rodrigues JM, Queiroz MJRP, Almeida BG, et al. Development of Thermo- and pH-sensitive liposomal magnetic carriers for new potential antitumor Thienopyridine derivatives. Materials (Basel). 2022;**15**(5):1737. DOI: 10.3390/ma15051737

[72] Trilli J, Caramazza L, Paolicelli P, Casadei MA, Liberti M, Apollonio F, et al. The impact of bilayer rigidity on the release from Magnetoliposomes vesicles controlled by PEMFs. Pharmaceutics. 2021;**13**(10):1712. DOI: 10.3390/pharmaceutics13101712

Chapter 4

Perspective Chapter: Nose-to-Brain Drug Delivery through Liposomes - Recent Applications

Abdul Hafeez and Shazia Afzal Usmani

Abstract

Diseases related to the brain are causing a huge problem worldwide. Different drug formulations are available for the management of brain-related disorders, but due to less drug availability for the brain and non-specificity, it becomes difficult to completely cure life-threatening brain disorders. The blood-brain barrier (BBB) restricts the entry of drug molecules/drug-loaded carriers because of the presence of various efflux transporters and drug inactivating enzymes. Researchers have identified an intranasal route for direct delivery to the brain, bypassing BBB. Nanotechnology-enabled lipid-based drug carrier systems have shown potential for the management of brain diseases through nose-to-brain delivery. Liposomes are the most extensively investigated carrier systems because of biocompatibility, controlled release characteristics, easy surface modification, and biodegradability. This chapter highlights the important aspects of nose-to-brain delivery and strategies for enhancing the availability of drugs through liposomes in the management of different brain-related diseases.

Keywords: liposomes, nanotechnology, brain tumor, brain delivery, Parkinson's disease, targeted delivery

1. Introduction

The diseases associated with the central nervous system (CNS) are continuously increasing in the populations worldwide in the last couple of decades. CNS disorders substantially contribute to the loss of health and social challenges across the lifespan of human beings. The CNS diseases causing numerous problems globally include Alzheimer's disease (AD), brain tumor, bipolar disorders, epilepsy, depression, Down's syndrome, Huntington's disease, Parkinson's disease (PD), multiple sclerosis, and schizophrenia [1, 2]. The major problem in the management of the mentioned disorders is the non-accessibility of most of the therapeutic compounds in the desired concentrations. The major hurdle for the entry of active pharmaceutical ingredients into the brain is the presence of blood-brain barrier (BBB), which separates the brain from the blood. The non-permeable nature of BBB is due to the presence of tight endothelial junctions supported by astrocytes and pericytes. Small lipid-soluble drug molecules can enter the brain through BBB and all large molecular weight drugs cannot enter the brain. Other factors responsible for nonentry of drugs into the brain are the presence of efflux transporters and drug inactivating enzymes onto the surface of BBB. P-glycoprotein is the most abundant efflux transporter, causing the non-availability of drug molecules into brain tissues. It becomes difficult for approximately 98% of drug candidates to enter into the brain tissues [3–6].

Various strategies have been investigated to facilitate the entry of drug molecules/ drug-loaded nanocarriers into the brain. It is categorized into invasive and non-invasive approaches [7]. Invasive approaches include intracerebral implants, BBB disruption, and intraventricular infusion, and these techniques are generally used during severe or emergency situations because of technical procedures and hazardous effects. Noninvasive approaches include delivery of drugs through different routes, such as oral, transdermal, and intranasal administration. These routes take advantage of the endogenous system present in the body that transports various nutrients to the brain [8]. Drugs are generally incorporated or attached to a carrier system that transports them through BBB in high concentrations. The intranasal drug delivery route has gained great interest in the last decade because of the direct access of compounds to the brain through olfactory and trigeminal nerves bypassing BBB. This route has other advantages like easy administration, bypassing hepatic metabolism, higher availability of drugs into brain tissues, patient compliance, and reduced adverse effects related to systemic exposure [9, 10]. It has been established now through various studies that this route has more potential in enhancing drug levels in the brain when compared to intravenous administration. The enhanced delivery into the brain has been supported by different preclinical and clinical investigations [11–15].

Pharmaceutical nanotechnology deals with studies related to nanostructures that can be utilized for the delivery of drugs. These nanostructures carry the drugs and can easily move through different biological barriers. The nanostructures can also be tailored to deliver the drugs at specific locations in the body by employing active and passive targeting approaches [16, 17]. Different nanocarriers are liposomes, ethosomes, polymeric nanoparticles, niosomes, solid lipid nanoparticles, micelles, silver nanoparticles nanostructured lipid carriers, carbon nanotubes, nanoemulsions, dendrimers, and gold nanoparticles [18, 19]. Encapsulation/entrapment of drug molecules in the mentioned carrier systems improve solubility, protection from the biological environment, and enhanced accumulation in the brain. In recent times, the intranasal route has been investigated for direct delivery to the brain by incorporating drug molecules in a variety of nanocarriers [20, 21]. Among the mentioned nanostructures, a significant amount of investigation has been centralized on liposomes. Liposomes consist of phospholipids with cholesterol. The components of liposomes make them biocompatible, less toxic, and biodegradable. Liposomes can hold hydrophilic as well as hydrophobic drug candidates into its inner and outer structures, respectively. The surface of liposomes can also be modified by different ligands for active drug targeting. This chapter summarizes the innovative approaches employed for the management of brain disorders through liposome-based nose-to-brain drug delivery [22, 23].

2. Anatomical and physiological aspects of nasal cavity

The primary functions of the nasal cavity are smelling, breathing, filtration of air, and protection. The nasal route, which starts from the nasal vestibule (nasal valve) till the nasopharynx, has a length of approximately 12–14 cm. The space between the human skull base and the roof of mouth filled by nasal cavity. Mucus layer and ciliary hair structures are found in the nasal cavity and help in trapping foreign particulate matters and pathogenic microorganisms. The total volume of the human nasal cavity is in between 15 and 20 ml with a total surface area of approximately 155 cm^2. The human nasal cavity is divided into the nasal vestibule, olfactory area, and respiratory region [24, 25].

Nasal vestibular part is the dilated area situated just after the nostrils. This part has the smallest surface area as compared to other parts of the nasal cavity. It does not have much significance in drug absorption and transport. The respiratory region of the nasal cavity, which is the largest segment with a large surface area (due to the presence of a large number of microvilli) of nasal cavity helps in the passage of air into the respiratory system. Each nostril's respiratory part consists of four conchae called turbinate bones and is covered by the mucosa of the nasal cavity [26]. Meatuses are present beneath the conchae and have connections till paranasal sinuses. The high vascularity and large surface area makes this section significant for drug absorption and transport. The presence of trigeminal nerves in this area has been investigated as a potential route for the direct entry of drug molecules into brain tissues. The olfactory area is placed in the deeper and upper part of the nasal cavity beneath the cribriform plate (horizontal bone). It helps in the processing of sensory information related to smell. In this area, olfactory neurons connect directly to olfactory bulb area of the brain. This target (olfactory neurons) in conjunction with the trigeminal route help has enhanced the uptake of drug/nanocarriers directly into CNS [27].

The rate of diffusion of drug formulations through the mucus layer and clearance rate from the nasal cavity is influenced by physical and chemical characteristics of polymer/excipient type, solvent system, particle size, shape, and surface charge. In adults, nasal secretions have pH in between 5.5 and 6.5 and contain different types of enzymes. The presence of enzymes deactivates different harmful substances entering from the outside environment. Drugs and polymers/additives can affect the functions of the ciliary structures of the nasal cavity. Rhinitis and nasal polyposis can also hamper the ciliary functioning and nasal absorption of drug molecules [28, 29].

3. Factors affecting drug diffusion from nose-to-brain

The environmental and physiological conditions of the nasal cavity contribute majorly to transportation of drug/carrier systems through nasal mucosa either into the systemic circulation or directly into the brain. The presence of drug-metabolizing enzymes, pH conditions, and tonicity characteristics of nasal secretions may severely affect the fate of drug molecules *in vivo* [30]. The different physicochemical factors related to drug molecule/drug formulation that can affect nasal transport are molecular weight, partition coefficient, degree of ionization, physical state of dosage form, viscosity, formulation pH, formulation osmolarity, and particle size [31]. It is reported that nasal absorption of drug molecules falls sharply if molecular weight exceeds beyond 1000 Da. Nasal absorption is significantly affected by the drug's lipophilicity and molecules with high lipophilic character are considered suitable for nasal delivery. In general, unionized molecules can traverse easily through the nasal barrier due to nonpolar characteristics [32, 33]. Intranasal delivery can be achieved by different states of formulations, such as liquid, powdered, and semisolids, but most of the formulations are developed in a liquid state because of easy administration and uniform distribution over the surface of the nasal cavity. It is desired to incorporate viscosity-enhancing agents and mucoadhesive materials in the formulation to prolong the residence time of formulation in the nasal cavity [34–36].

Formulation pH also affects significantly with respect to ionization of drug, stability and might cause irritation of nasal mucosa if not adjusted properly. The osmolarity of the formulation can affect ciliary movement that can affect drug permeation and transport through the nasal barrier. The particle size of nanocarrier systems greatly influences the deposition and diffusion characteristics in the nasal cavity. It is generally desirable to have particle size of less than 200 nm for effective permeation and drug release behavior. Administered dose, volume, and administration device also affect the extent of nanocarrier localization and deposition in the nasal cavity [37]. Permeation enhancers can be incorporated into formulations to enhance diffusion through the nasal epithelium. These enhancers must have suitable characteristics such as nonirritating, nonallergic, nontoxic, and not causing any changes in the cells of nasal epithelium. Sodium deoxycholate, sodium taurocholate, sodium taurodihydrofusidate, sodium dodecyl sulfate, and polyoxyethylene-9-lauryl ether are the most commonly investigated permeation enhancers for nasal drug delivery [38].

4. Liposome-based nose-to-brain drug delivery applications

Nanotechnology deals with structures that have size ranges in nanometers. Methods for the preparation of nanocarriers govern the size, shape, encapsulation, and stability characteristics. Nose-to-brain route requires specific size requirements (less than 200 nm) for efficient drug delivery. Liposomes are lipid-based vesicular systems designed for encapsulation of hydrophilic and lipophilic drug molecules. Hydrophilic drug molecules can be incorporated into the inner aqueous compartment of liposomes, while lipophilic drugs in the phospholipid bilayer structure. The availability of biocompatible and biodegradable lipids makes this vesicular system suitable for therapeutic applications [22, 23, 39]. Nose-to-brain approaches have been utilized and reported through liposomes by researchers across the world for the management of different CNS disorders. Passive and active targeting strategies have been adopted to enhance the accumulation of drugs into brain tissues through liposomes. Passive strategy is based on the physiological processes followed by hormones and neurotransmitters of the human body. Active targeting involves the attachment of a ligand onto the liposomal surface, which specifically binds to a specific type of cells in the brain. Stimuli-sensitive liposomal formulations are also developed based on pH change, temperature, and other factors [40, 41].

Recent studies employing liposomal formulations through the intranasal route for the management of brain diseases are briefed herein and summarized in **Table 1** with major outcomes.

4.1 Brain cancer

Cancers are the most difficult disease to treat because variable nature of cancerous cells and high resistance to different drug candidates. Brain cancer is the most challenging aspect of therapeutics due to non-accessibility of drugs. The effectiveness of conventional chemotherapy is limited due to the non-specificity and toxicity of anticancer drugs [55]. In brain tumor situations, formulations first must overcome the BBB. Several researchers have developed liposome-based intranasal formulations

Drug(s) name	Drug category/ disease evaluation	Major outcome	References
Lomustine (LM) and *n*-propyl gallate (NPG)	Brain cancer	Liposomal size of ~127 nm with a sustained release pattern, enhanced nasal permeation, and cell killing activity against *in vitro* cancer cell lines were obtained.	[42]
Curcumin	Anticancer/anti-inflammatory/ antioxidant	The obtained liposomal size was between 100.2 and 150 nm. The optimized formulation exhibited controlled release characteristics with enhanced accumulation of curcumin in the brain via intranasal route when compared to curcumin solution.	[43]
Rivastigmine tartrate	Alzheimer's disease	Liposomal size with ell-penetrating peptide was found to be 178.9 ± 11.7 nm with an entrapment efficiency of ~30%. In vivo intranasal data revealed enhanced accumulation of rivastigmine tartrate in the cortex and hippocampus when compared to intravenous administration.	[44]
Galanthamine hydrobromide	Alzheimer's disease	Flexible liposomes showed size, zeta potential, and entrapment efficiency of 112 ± 8 nm, −49.2 ± 0.7 mV, and 83.6 ± 1.8%, respectively. More anti-acetylcholinesterase activity and higher brain concentration were found with developed intranasal liposomes in comparison to oral administration.	[45]
Donepezil	Alzheimer's disease	Liposomal formulation exhibited size of 102 ± 3.3 nm with an encapsulation efficiency of 84.91% ± 3.31%. A high drug concentration of the drug in the brain was found after intranasal administration through liposomes.	[46]
Hydroxy-α-Sanshool	Alzheimer's disease	The size obtained was 181.77 nm with PDI value of 0.207. The developed liposomal formulation was found to be nontoxic to the nasal mucosa of mouse and significantly improved learning memory deficits of the disease.	[47]
Glial cell line-derived neurotrophic factor (GDNF)	Parkinson's disease	Brain levels improved significantly within 1 h after a single dose (50-μg) of GDNF delivered by liposomal formulation through intranasal administration compared to GDNF delivered by phosphate buffer saline solution.	[48]
Risperidone	Schizophrenia	Vesicular size obtained was between 90 and100 nm with a PDI value of less than 0.5. The amount of risperidone was found to be high in the brain in comparison to plasma through intranasal delivery, depicting preferential transport to the brain.	[49]

Drug(s) name	Drug category/ disease evaluation	Major outcome	References
Quetiapine fumarate	Schizophrenia	The average liposomal size obtained was 152.2 nm with a zeta potential value of 24.7 mV. A higher concentration of drug was observed in the brain of albino mice from liposomal dispersion when compared to simple dispersion of drug.	[50]
Lamotrigine	Epilepsy	Optimized liposomal formulation exhibited a size of 88.90 ± 1.56 nm with an entrapment efficiency of 68.75% ± 0.02%. Significantly high drug permeation was obtained with the liposomal formulation in comparison to simple dispersion.	[51]
Valproic acid	Epilepsy	Liposomal size obtained was in between 90 and 210 nm with entrapment efficiency ranging in between 60% and 85%. Pharmacokinetic studies showed a higher amount of drug in the brain than plasma after intranasal administration.	[52]
Tissue plasminogen activator	Ischemic stroke	Suitable entrapment efficiency with the desired size, sustained release characteristics and proteolytic activity showed the potential of nanoliposomes in the management of cardiovascular conditions.	[53]
Basic fibroblast growth factor (bFGF)	Ischemic stroke	bFGF-loaded liposomes showed the size of 106 ± 9.84 nm, PDI value of <0.2, and zeta potential value of <−15 mV. Liposomal formulation exhibited the highest reduction in infarcted volume when compared to bFGF solution.	[54]

Table 1.
Applications of intranasally delivered drug-loaded liposomes with major outcomes.

for encapsulation of a variety of anticancer drugs. In a very recent study, Katona et al. formulated LM and NPG-loaded liposomes by a novel direct pouring method for targeting glioblastoma multiforme via nose-to-brain route. Phosphatidylcholine and cholesterol were utilized for the preparation of liposomes. The optimized liposomal formulation encapsulated with both drugs exhibited a suitable *Z*-average of ~127 nm, size distribution (PDI value of 0.142 ± 0.009), zeta potential value of -34 ± 1.7 mV, and high encapsulation efficiency of 63.57% ± 1.3% for NPG and 73.45% ± 2.2% of LM, respectively. These results demonstrated the suitability of an optimized formulation for nose-to-brain drug delivery. The dialysis-based release method was adopted and results indicated a sustained release pattern from the optimized liposomal formulation. Nasal permeation studies revealed higher permeation of drugs from the optimized liposomal formulation in comparison to the suspension of drugs. MTT assays of the developed formulation were also performed on murine embryonic fibroblast (NIH/3T3), glioblastoma (U87), and ovarian (A2780) cancer cell lines. The results of *in vitro* cancer cell line indicated a reduction in cancerous cells of all studied types [42].

Phytoconstituents, such as curcumin, a polyphenolic compound obtained from the rhizomes of Curcuma longa and show anti-inflammatory and antioxidant characteristics. Curcumin has potential in the management of brain cancer and other neurodegenerative disorders [56]. Studies have been conducted to enhance the availability of curcumin by incorporation into liposomes through nose-to-brain delivery. In a study, a mucoadhesive liposomal formulation of curcumin was developed and optimized for nasal delivery. The liposomes were formulated by solvent dispersion method employing cholesterol and soya lecithin as lipid bilayer forming material and xanthan gum for mucoadhesion. The vesicular size was found to be between 100.2 and 150 nm. The optimized formulation showed good stability and controlled/sustained release characteristics. The liposomal formulation was also found nontoxic to the nasal mucosa of rats. *In vivo* studies in rats revealed higher curcumin concentration (1240 ng) in the brain when compared to free drug solution (65 ng) when administered intranasally. The authors concluded the potential of curcumin liposomes with xanthan gum coating for enhancement of curcumin concentrations in the brain via the intranasal route [43].

4.2 Alzheimer's disease

AD leads to a decline in thinking, memory, learning, and language capacity. FDA-approved drugs used for AD are donepezil, memantine, galanthamine, and rivastigmine [57]. Yang et al. formulated rivastigmine tartrate-loaded liposomes with ell-penetrating peptide modification. The developed liposomes showed uniform sizes and shapes. A mean diameter of 166.3 ± 17.4 nm was found for simple liposomes and 178.9 ± 11.7 nm with ell-penetrating peptide-modified liposomes with low PDI values. The entrapment efficiency of slightly more than 30% was found for both types of liposomes. The results exhibited that liposomes, especially the ell-penetrating peptide enhanced the permeability through *in vitro* murine brain endothelial cells model. Intranasal administration of rivastigmine in solution and liposomal form demonstrated improvement of rivastigmine distribution and retention in CNS areas, particularly in the cortex and hippocampus, which are the most affected regions in AD when compared to intravenous administration. Developed liposomal formulations exhibited safety potential toward nasal mucosa. The authors concluded the potential of intranasal rivastigmine liposomes with ell-penetrating peptide improved brain delivery with enhancement in pharmacodynamic activity [44]. In another report, galanthamine hydrobromide-loaded flexible liposomes were formulated by the thin film homogenization method with some modification. Liposomal components used were soya phosphatidylcholine and cholesterol. Propylene glycol was used as an edge activator. The average size of drug-loaded flexible liposomes was found to be 112 ± 8 nm with a zeta potential of −49.2 ± 0.7 mV. This negative charge indicated the repulsive power of liposomal vesicles in the liposomal dispersion, which is important for long-term stability. The entrapment efficiency was found to be 83.6% ± 1.8%. The inhibition of acetylcholinesterase was studied by using brain homogenates of rats as an enzyme resource. The microdialysis technique was employed to investigate the pharmacokinetic characteristics of galanthamine hydrobromide in rat brain. It was found that inhibition of acetylcholinesterase was more by intranasal administration when compared to oral administration. The C_{max}, $AUC_{0\rightarrow 10}$ from intranasal administration of galanthamine hydrobromide-loaded liposomes were 3.52, 3.36 times more than those through oral administration of galanthamine hydrobromide. The authors further reported the safety of developed liposomes tested against PC-12 cells [45]. Al Asmari et al. developed liposomes of donepezil using cholesterol, 1,2-distearyl-sn-glycero-3-phosphocholine, and polyethylene glycol by thin film hydration method. The liposomal size was consistent with 102 ± 3.3 nm with proper shape and encapsulation efficiency of 84.91% ± 3.31%. The developed formulation exhibited sustained release behavior. It has found high drug concentration in plasma and brain after intranasal administration. Histopathological examination revealed safety for the developed liposomal formulation of donepezil [46].

In a very recent study, hydroxy-α-sanshool was incorporated into liposomes. This drug helps in cognitive dysfunction. Liposomes were fabricated by a thin film dispersion technique using cholesterol and soya lecithin. Liposomal formulations exhibited a vesicle size of 181.77 nm, PDI value of 0.207, and zeta potential of − 53.8 mV with good stability. Drug release studies revealed slow and consistent release following Higuchi kinetics. Highly drug concentration was found in plasma and brain after intranasal administration. Developed liposomes were not toxic to the mouse nasal mucosa and effectively improved learning memory deficits induced by D-galactose and protected mouse neuronal cells of the hippocampus. The authors concluded that these hydroxy-α-sanshool liposomes might be used for the management of AD [47].

4.3 Parkinson's disease

PD is caused by degenerative effects on dopamine regulating neurons in the area of substantia nigra pars compacta. Levodopa is most commonly a prodrug for the management of PD but its efflux by P-gp and enzymes diminishes its activity. GDNF has shown significant neuroprotective effects on substantia nigra neurons in the 6-hydroxydopamine rat model of PD [58]. GDNF cationic liposomes were prepared by using dioleoylphosphatidylcholine, stearylamine, and cholesterol. Enzyme-linked immunosorbent assay was used to determine brain levels of GDNF and distribution to target areas (striatum and substantia nigra) after intranasal administration at different time intervals. Brain levels enhanced significantly within 1 h after a single dose (50-μg) of GDNF incorporated into the liposomal formulation. In the second study, different doses (10–150 μg) of GDNF in phosphate buffer saline solution were administered. Liposomal formulation delivered 10-fold more amount of GDNF to the brain than phosphate buffer saline. The results suggested the potential of liposomes for enhanced delivery of GDNF in the brain tissues for the management of PD after intranasal administration [48].

4.4 Schizophrenia

Schizophrenia results in psychosis and may affect all aspects of life, including social, educational, personal, family, and occupational functioning. Schizophrenia affects approximately 1 in 300 people worldwide. A variety of drugs are available for the management of this disease but due to non-availability in the right amount in the brain tissue is the major issue in the treatment of this problem [59, 60]. Narayan et al. developed risperidone liposomes employing the method of thin film hydration. Design expert software was used to optimize formulation components. The optimized liposomal surface was modified by stearylamine and MPEG-DSPE coating for the enhancement of brain penetration. The mean vesicular size of liposomes was obtained between 90 and 100 nm with a polydispersity index of less than 0.5 with entrapment efficiency ranging from 50% to 60% and maximum drug entrapment was found with functionalized liposomes. Transmission electron micrographs revealed smooth and bilayer structures. A prolonged and controlled release behavior was obtained with a developed liposomal formulation. It was further established through *in vivo* studies that risperidone concentration was high in the brain in comparison to plasma from liposomal formulation through intranasal delivery [49]. In another report, quetiapine fumarate was incorporated in liposomal vesicles. Sheep nasal membrane diffusion was compared for simple dispersion and liposomal dispersion of quetiapine fumarate. Simple dispersion was prepared using a colloid mill in SNF pH 6.8. Liposomes of quetiapine fumarate were manufactured by the thin lipid film hydration method. The average particular size from simple dispersion obtained was 139.6 nm with a zeta potential of 32.1 mV. The average vesicular size from liposomal dispersion obtained was 152.2 nm with a zeta potential of 24.7 mV. The drug diffusion from liposomal dispersion was found higher (32.61 ± 1.70) with a high permeability coefficient of 4.1334 ± 0.7321 ($\times 10^{-5}$ cm/s). In vivo studies revealed a higher amount of quetiapine fumarate in the brain from liposomal dispersion in comparison to simple dispersion [50].

4.5 Epilepsy

Epilepsy is characterized by repeated and recurrent seizures involving involuntary movement of the whole body or part. These symptoms are due to electrical discharges in excess from cortical neurons. Management of epilepsy is difficult due to less access to drugs in brain tissues. Nanotechnological developments of already approved drugs have been found to enhance drug concentrations in the brain [61]. Praveen et al. developed nanoliposomes of lamotrigine for the management of seizures. The liposomes were prepared by thin film hydration method employing phospholipid as phospholipon 90G, vesicle stabilizer as cholesterol, and surfactant as tween 80. Plackett-Burman's design was used to optimize the liposomal formulation. Optimized formulation showed the vesicular size of 88.90 ± 1.56 nm with polydispersity index of 0.247 ± 0.04, entrapment efficiency of 68.75% ± 0.02%, and *in vitro* drug release of 79.41% ± 1.15%. These results were in close agreement with predicted responses. The optimized formulation was found to be stable at different storage temperatures. Nasal mucosa (goat) permeation studies showed higher drug permeation from liposomes (72.45% ± 2.15%) in comparison to simple suspension (13.27% ± 1.17%) after 12 h. Confocal laser scanning micrographs revealed higher fluorescence intensity in the deeper layer of the nasal mucosa. The results suggested the high potential of the liposomal system for enhanced delivery of lamotrigine through the intranasal route [51]. In a recent study, valproic acid was incorporated into liposomes utilizing phosphatidylcholine and cholesterol by the method of thin film hydration. The mean vesicular size of optimized liposomes was obtained between 90 and 210 nm with a low polydispersity index of less than 0.5. The entrapment efficiency obtained was between 60% and 85%. Transmission electron microscopy examination revealed the spherical shape of liposomes. Permeation studies involving sheep's nasal mucosa exhibited higher permeation of valproic acid from liposomes in comparison to control samples. Animal studies revealed a higher concentration of drug in the brain than plasma after administration through the intranasal route [52].

4.6 Ischemic stroke

Stroke is the prevalent cause of death globally. Ischemic stroke is caused by blockage or narrowing of a blood vessel supplying blood to the brain. Interruption of glucose and oxygen supply leads to a reduction in the production of ATP, causing energy failure and irregularities in ion homeostasis. Recombinant tissue plasminogen activator (rt-PA) is approved by the FDA for the management of ischemic stroke. It acts by dissolving the blood clot in cerebral vessels with the restoration of blood flow, which results in the protection of brain tissue. The short half-life (2–6 minutes) causes problem in the management of the disease and requires nanotechnological carrier system interventions [62, 63]. In a recent study, nanoliposomes of tissue plasminogen activators have been reported for improvement of the thrombolytic activity. The results suggested the stability of nanoliposomes with no aggregation when stored at 4°C. A desirable entrapment efficiency, zeta potential, proteolytic activity, and sustained *in vitro* release characteristics were obtained. The authors suggested the use of developed nanoliposomes of tissue plasminogen activators, which could be used in the management of cardiovascular diseases [53]. Another therapeutic basic bFGF has the potential to protect against ischemic stroke. Zhao et al. reported nanoliposomes of bFGF by the technique of water-in-water emulsion followed by freeze-drying. The average vesicular sizes of blank and bFGF-loaded nanoliposomes obtained were 106 ± 9.84, 128 ± 7.65 nm, respectively, with low polydispersity index (<0.2). Negative zeta potential values (<-15 mV) were observed for both types of liposomes. Western blotting was conducted to analyze the bFGF levels in the olfactory bulb, hippocampus, pallium, and striatum after intranasal administration. Intranasal administration of bFGF-loaded nanoliposomes enhanced the concentration of bFGF in pallium and hippocampus. After comparison with intravenous delivery, it was found that intranasal delivery is superior in delivering the bFGF into different brain areas. Further results like recovery of neurological function strengthened the suitability of nanoliposomes of bFGF through intranasal administration. Therapeutic efficacy was determined after ischemia-reperfusion injury followed by the determination of neurological deficit scores. The bFGF-loaded nanoliposomes exhibited higher scores in treated animals than bFGF solution. Liposomal treatment resulted in the highest reduction in the infarcted volume. The authors concluded that intranasal bFGF-loaded liposomal therapy was effective and was able to enhance the recovery effect of bFGF after ischemia-reperfusion injury [54].

5. Conclusions

Pharmaceutical nanocarriers are successfully being evaluated for their potential through intranasal delivery in the improvement of characteristics of already approved molecules and new chemical entities as well as used for brain diseases [64]. Liposomes have attracted researchers globally due to their excellent biocompatible and biodegradable characteristics. A variety of research works have been reported for the delivery of drugs encapsulated in liposomes through the intranasal route [42–44]. Several studies have been reported for intranasal liposomes for the management of brain diseases, such as brain cancer, AD, PD, schizophrenia, epilepsy, and ischemic stroke. Most of the optimization studies included the effect of phospholipid concentration, cholesterol amount, process parameters on the size, encapsulation efficiency, zeta potential, and release characteristics of liposomes. Optimized formulations were investigated for the availability of the drug in the brain and its pharmacological effect after intranasal administration. Research findings revealed favorable physicochemical characteristics of the drug after incorporation into liposomes. Intranasal liposomal formulations exhibited enhanced uptake into the brain with enhanced activity in the concerned brain disease. Results suggested the potential of intranasal liposomal formulations for the management of brain diseases. A more mechanistic approach is needed for the identification of drug transport to brain areas.

Acknowledgements

The authors are thankful to the Chancellor, Integral University, Lucknow, India for his continuous encouragement, supervision, and valuable suggestions at all stages of this chapter. The authors are grateful to the Faculty of Pharmacy, Integral University for providing necessary facilities related to this work. The authors are also grateful to the research cell, Integral University for continuous guidance and support.

Conflict of interest

The authors declare no conflict of interest.

Author details

Abdul Hafeez* and Shazia Afzal Usmani
Faculty of Pharmacy, Integral University, Lucknow, India

*Address all correspondence to: abdulhafeez@iul.ac.in

References

[1] Catalá-López F, Hutton B, Driver JA, Page MJ, Ridao M, Valderas JM, et al. Cancer and central nervous system disorders: protocol for an umbrella review of systematic reviews and updated meta-analyses of observational studies. Systematic Reviews. 2017;**6**(1):69. DOI: 10.1186/s13643-017-0466-y

[2] Organization WH. Neurological Disorders Affect Millions Globally: WHO report. World Health Organization; Switzerland. 2007. Available from: http://www.who.int/mental_health/neurology/neurological_disorders_report_web.pdf

[3] Agrawal M, Ajazuddin TDK, Saraf S, Saraf S, Antimisiaris SG, Mourtas S, et al. Recent advancements in liposomes targeting strategies to cross blood-brain barrier (BBB) for the treatment of Alzheimer's disease. Journal of Controlled Release. 2017;**260**:61-77. DOI: 10.1016/j.jconrel.2017.05.019

[4] Bourganis V, Kammona O, Alexopoulos A, Kiparissides C. Recent advances in carrier mediated nose-to-brain delivery of pharmaceutics. European Journal of Pharmaceutics and Biopharmaceutics. 2018;**128**:337-362. DOI: 10.1016/j.ejpb.2018.05.009

[5] Montesinos R. Liposomal drug delivery to the central nervous system. In: Catala A, editor. Liposomes. London: IntechOpen; 2017. DOI: 10.5772/intechopen.70055

[6] Samaridou E, Alonso MJ. Nose-to-brain peptide delivery - the potential of nanotechnology. Bioorganic & Medicinal Chemistry 2018;**26**(10):2888-2905. DOI: 10.1016/j.bmc.2017.11.001. Epub 2017 Nov 4. PMID: 29170026

[7] Banks WA. From blood-brain barrier to blood-brain interface: new opportunities for CNS drug delivery. Nature Reviews Drug Discovery 2016;**15**(4):275-292. DOI: 10.1038/nrd.2015.21. Epub 2016 Jan 22. PMID: 26794270

[8] Joshi S, Ergin A, Wang M, Reif R, Zhang J, Bruce JN, et al. Inconsistent blood brain barrier disruption by intraarterial mannitol in rabbits: implications for chemotherapy. Journal of Neuro-Oncology. 2011;**104**(1):11-19. DOI: 10.1007/s11060-010-0466-4

[9] Rodriguez A, Tatter SB, Debinski W. Neurosurgical techniques for disruption of the blood-brain barrier for glioblastoma treatment. Pharmaceutics. 2015;**7**(3):175-187. Published 2015 Aug 3. DOI: 10.3390/pharmaceutics7030175

[10] Gaillard PJ, Appeldoorn CC, Rip J, Dorland R, van der Pol SM, Kooij G, et al. Enhanced brain delivery of liposomal methylprednisolone improved therapeutic efficacy in a model of neuroinflammation. Journal of Controlled Release. 2012;**164**(3):364-369. DOI: 10.1016/j.jconrel.2012.06.022

[11] Khan AR, Liu M, Khan MW, Zhai G. Progress in brain targeting drug delivery system by nasal route. Journal of Controlled Release. 2017;**268**:364-389. DOI: 10.1016/j.jconrel.2017.09.001

[12] Born J, Lange T, Kern W, McGregor GP, Bickel U, Fehm HL. Sniffing neuropeptides: a transnasal approach to the human brain. Nature Neuroscience. 2002;**5**(6):514-516. DOI: 10.1038/nn849

[13] de la Monte SM. Intranasal insulin therapy for cognitive impairment and

neurodegeneration: current state of the art. Expert Opinion on Drug Delivery. 2013;**10**(12):1699-1709. DOI: 10.1517/17425247.2013.856877

[14] Hallschmid M. Intranasal insulin for Alzheimer's disease. CNS Drugs. 2021;**35**(1):21-37. DOI: 10.1007/s40263-020-00781-x

[15] Muntimadugu E, Dhommati R, Jain A, Challa VG, Shaheen M, Khan W. Intranasal delivery of nanoparticle encapsulated tarenflurbil: a potential brain targeting strategy for Alzheimer's disease. European Journal of Pharmaceutical Sciences. 2016;**92**:224-234. DOI: 10.1016/j.ejps.2016.05.012

[16] Nakamura T, Harashima H. Integration of nano drug-delivery system with cancer immunotherapy. Therapeutic Delivery. 2017;**8**(11):987-1000. DOI: 10.4155/tde-2017-0071

[17] De Jong WH, Borm PJ. Drug delivery and nanoparticles: applications and hazards. International Journal of Nanomedicine. 2008;**3**(2):133-149. DOI: 10.2147/ijn.s596

[18] Hamid R, Manzoor I. Nanomedicines: Nano based drug delivery systems challenges and opportunities. In: Akram M, editor. Alternative Medicine – Update. London: IntechOpen; 2020. DOI: 10.5772/intechopen.94353

[19] Shi J, Votruba AR, Farokhzad OC, Langer R. Nanotechnology in drug delivery and tissue engineering: from discovery to applications. Nano Letters. 2010;**10**(9):3223-3230. DOI: 10.1021/nl102184c

[20] Wang Z, Xiong G, Tsang WC, Schätzlein AG, Uchegbu IF. Nose-to-brain delivery. Journal of Pharmacology and Experimental Therapeutics 2019;**370**(3):593-601. DOI: 10.1124/jpet.119.258152. Epub 2019 May 24. PMID: 31126978

[21] Kashyap K, Shukla R. Drug delivery and targeting to the brain through nasal route: mechanisms, applications and challenges. Current Drug Delivery. 2019;**16**(10):887-901. DOI: 10.2174/1567201816666191029122740

[22] Li M, Du C, Guo N, Teng Y, Meng X, Sun H, et al. Composition design and medical application of liposomes. European Journal of Medicinal Chemistry. 2019;**164**:640-653. DOI: 10.1016/j.ejmech.2019.01.007

[23] Guimarães D, Cavaco-Paulo A, Nogueira E. Design of liposomes as drug delivery system for therapeutic applications. International Journal of Pharmaceutics. 2021;**601**:120571. DOI: 10.1016/j.ijpharm.2021.120571

[24] Sahin-Yilmaz A, Naclerio RM. Anatomy and physiology of the upper airway. Proceedings of the American Thoracic Society. 2011;**8**(1):31-39. DOI: 10.1513/pats.201007-050RN

[25] Watelet JB, Van Cauwenberge P. Applied anatomy and physiology of the nose and paranasal sinuses. Allergy. 1999;**54**(Suppl. 57):14-25. DOI: 10.1111/j.1398-9995.1999.tb04402.x

[26] Jones N. The nose and paranasal sinuses physiology and anatomy. Advanced Drug Delivery Reviews. 2001;**51**(1-3):5-19. DOI: 10.1016/s0169-409x(01)00172-7

[27] Patel RG. Nasal anatomy and function. Facial Plastic Surgery. 2017;**33**(1):3-8. DOI: 10.1055/s-0036-1597950 Epub 2017 Feb 22

[28] Gizurarson S. Anatomical and histological factors affecting intranasal

drug and vaccine delivery. Current Drug Delivery. 2012;**9**(6):566-582. DOI: 10.2174/156720112803529828

[29] Costa C, Moreira JN, Amaral MH, Sousa Lobo JM, Silva AC. Nose-to-brain delivery of lipid-based nanosystems for epileptic seizures and anxiety crisis. Journal of Controlled Release. 2019;**295**:187-200. DOI: 10.1016/j.jconrel.2018.12.049

[30] Inoue D. Development of prediction system for drug absorption after intranasal administration incorporating physiologic functions of nose -estimation of in vivo drug permeation through nasal mucosa using in vitro membrane permeability. Yakugaku Zasshi. 2021;**141**(11):1235-1240. Japanese. DOI: 10.1248/yakushi.21-00151

[31] Campbell C, Morimoto BH, Nenciu D, Fox AW. Drug development of intranasally delivered peptides. Therapeutic Delivery. 2012;**3**(4):557-568. DOI: 10.4155/tde.12.12

[32] Hussain AA. Intranasal drug delivery. Advanced Drug Delivery Reviews. 1998;**29**(1-2):39-49. DOI: 10.1016/s0169-409x(97)00060-4

[33] Arora P, Sharma S, Garg S. Permeability issues in nasal drug delivery. Drug Discovery Today. 2002;**7**(18):967-975. DOI: 10.1016/s1359-6446(02)02452-2

[34] Agarwal V, Mishra B. Recent trends in drug delivery systems: intranasal drug delivery. Indian Journal of Experimental Biology. 1999;**37**(1):6-16

[35] Laffleur F, Bauer B. Progress in nasal drug delivery systems. International Journal of Pharmaceutics. 2021;**607**:120994. DOI: 10.1016/j.ijpharm.2021.120994

[36] Furubayashi T, Inoue D, Kamaguchi A, Higashi Y, Sakane T. Influence of formulation viscosity on drug absorption following nasal application in rats. Drug Metabolism and Pharmacokinetics. 2007;**22**(3):206-211. DOI: 10.2133/dmpk.22.206

[37] Dua R, Duncan M, Zia H, Needham TE. The influence of the enhancerdimyristoylphosphatidylglycerol and formulation factors on the nasal absorption of salmon calcitonin. Drug Delivery. 1998;**5**(2):127-134. DOI: 10.3109/10717549809031388

[38] Kim NA, Thapa R, Jeong SH, Bae HD, Maeng J, Lee K, et al. Enhanced intranasal insulin delivery by formulations and tumor protein-derived protein transduction domain as an absorption enhancer. Journal of Controlled Release. 2019;**294**:226-236. DOI: 10.1016/j.jconrel.2018.12.023

[39] Shah S, Dhawan V, Holm R, Nagarsenker MS, Perrie Y. Liposomes: advancements and innovation in the manufacturing process. Advanced Drug Delivery Reviews. 2020;**154-155**:102-122. DOI: 10.1016/j.addr.2020.07.002

[40] Dong X. Current strategies for brain drug delivery. Theranostics. 2018;**8**(6):1481-1493. DOI: 10.7150/thno.21254

[41] Xie J, Shen Z, Anraku Y, Kataoka K, Chen X. Nanomaterial-based blood-brain-barrier (BBB) crossing strategies. Biomaterials. 2019;**224**:119491. DOI: 10.1016/j.biomaterials.2019.119491

[42] Katona G, Sabir F, Sipos B, Naveed M, Schelz Z, Zupkó I, et al. Development of lomustine and n-propyl gallate co-encapsulated liposomes for targeting glioblastoma multiforme via intranasal administration.

Pharmaceutics. 2022;**14**(3):631-652. DOI: 10.3390/pharmaceutics14030631

[43] Samudre S, Tekade A, Thorve K, Jamodkar A, Parashar G, Chaudhari N. Xanthan gum coated mucoadhesive liposomes for efficient nose to brain delivery of curcumin. Drug Delivery Letters. 2015;**5**(3):201-207. DOI: 10.2174/2210303106666160120215857

[44] Yang ZZ, Zhang YQ, Wang ZZ, Wu K, Lou JN, Qi XR. Enhanced brain distribution and pharmacodynamics of rivastigmine by liposomes following intranasal administration. International Journal of Pharmaceutics. 2013;**452**(1-2):344-354. DOI: 10.1016/j.ijpharm.2013.05.009

[45] Li W, Zhou Y, Zhao N, Hao B, Wang X, Kong P. Pharmacokinetic behavior and efficiency of acetylcholinesterase inhibition in rat brain after intranasal administration of galanthamine hydrobromide loaded flexible liposomes. Environmental Toxicology and Pharmacology. 2012;**34**(2):272-279. DOI: 10.1016/j.etap.2012.04.012

[46] Al Asmari AK, Ullah Z, Tariq M, Fatani A. Preparation, characterization, and in vivo evaluation of intranasally administered liposomal formulation of donepezil. Drug Design, Development and Therapy. 2016;**10**:205-215. DOI: 10.2147/DDDT.S93937

[47] Li R, Lu F, Sun X, He L, Duan H, Peng W, et al. Development and in vivo evaluation of hydroxy-α-sanshool intranasal liposomes as a potential remedial treatment for Alzheimer's disease. International Journal of Nanomedicine. 2022;**17**:185-201. DOI: 10.2147/IJN.S339979

[48] Bender TS, Migliore MM, Campbell RB, John Gatley S, Waszczak BL. Intranasal administration of glial-derived neurotrophic factor (GDNF) rapidly and significantly increases whole-brain GDNF level in rats. Neuroscience. 2015;**303**:569-576. DOI: 10.1016/j.neuroscience.2015.07.016

[49] Narayan R, Singh M, Ranjan O, Nayak Y, Garg S, Shavi GV, et al. Development of risperidone liposomes for brain targeting through intranasal route. Life Sciences. 2016;**163**:38-45. DOI: 10.1016/j.lfs.2016.08.033

[50] Upadhyay P, Trivedi J, Pundarikakshudu K, Sheth N. Comparative study between simple and optimized liposomal dispersion of quetiapine fumarate for diffusion through nasal route. Drug Delivery. 2016;**23**(4):1214-1221. DOI: 10.3109/10717544.2015.1120364

[51] Praveen A, Aqil M, Imam SS, Ahad A, Moolakkadath T, Ahmad FJ. Lamotrigine encapsulated intra-nasal nanoliposome formulation for epilepsy treatment: formulation design, characterization and nasal toxicity study. Colloids and Surfaces. B, Biointerfaces. 2019;**174**:553-562. DOI: 10.1016/j.colsurfb.2018.11.025

[52] Yuwanda A, Surini S, Harahap Y, Jufri M. Study of valproic acid liposomes for delivery into the brain through an intranasal route. Heliyon. 2022;**8**(3):e09030. DOI: 10.1016/j.heliyon.2022.e09030

[53] Dubatouka K, Agabekov V. Preparation and characterization of tissue plasminogen activator-loaded liposomes. Soft Materials. 2022;**20**(3):358-363. DOI: 10.1080/1539445X.2021.2007128

[54] Zhao YZ, Lin M, Lin Q, Yang W, Yu XC, Tian FR, et al. Intranasal delivery of bFGF with nanoliposomes enhances

in vivo neuroprotection and neural injury recovery in a rodent stroke model. Journal of Controlled Release. 2016;**224**:165-175. DOI: 10.1016/j.jconrel.2016.01.017

[55] Shah V, Kochar P. Brain cancer: implication to disease, therapeutic strategies and tumor targeted drug delivery approaches. Recent Patents on Anti-Cancer Drug Discovery. 2018;**13**(1):70-85. DOI: 10.2174/1574892812666171129142023

[56] Kotha RR, Luthria DL. Curcumin: biological, pharmaceutical, nutraceutical, and analytical aspects. Molecules. 2019;**24**(16):2930. DOI: 10.3390/molecules24162930

[57] Khan S, Barve KH, Kumar MS. Recent advancements in pathogenesis, diagnostics and treatment of Alzheimer's disease. Current Neuropharmacology. 2020;**18**(11):1106-1125. DOI: 10.2174/1570159X18666200528142429

[58] Schneider RB, Iourinets J, Richard IH. Parkinson's disease psychosis: presentation, diagnosis and management. Neurodegenerative Disease Management. 2017;**7**(6):365-376. DOI: 10.2217/nmt-2017-0028

[59] Häfner H, an der Heiden W. Epidemiology of schizophrenia. Canadian Journal of Psychiatry. 1997;**42**(2):139-151. DOI: 10.1177/070674379704200204

[60] Bortolon C, Macgregor A, Capdevielle D, Raffard S. Apathy in schizophrenia: a review of neuropsychological and neuroanatomical studies. Neuropsychologia. 2018;**118**(Pt B):22-33. DOI: 10.1016/j.neuropsychologia.2017.09.033

[61] Manford M. Recent advances in epilepsy. Journal of Neurology. 2017;**264**(8):1811-1824. DOI: 10.1007/s00415-017-8394-2

[62] Iadecola C, Anrather J. Stroke research at a crossroad: asking the brain for directions. Nature Neuroscience. 2011;**14**(11):1363-1368. DOI: 10.1038/nn.2953

[63] Feske SK. Ischemic stroke. American Journal of Medicine. 2021;**134**(12):1457-1464. DOI: 10.1016/j.amjmed.2021.07.027

[64] Erdő F, Bors LA, Farkas D, Bajza Á, Gizurarson S. Evaluation of intranasal delivery route of drug administration for brain targeting. Brain Research Bulletin. 2018;**143**:155-170. DOI: 10.1016/j.brainresbull.2018.10.009

Section 2

Liposomes in Nanobiomedicine

Chapter 5

Perspective Chapter: Liposome Mediated Delivery of Immunotherapeutics for Cancer

Alessandra Iscaro, Faith H.N. Howard, Zidi Yang, Fern Jenkins and Munitta Muthana

Abstract

Tumors have complex properties that depend on interactions between epithelial cancer cells and the surrounding stromal compartment within the tumor microenvironment. In particular, immune infiltration plays a role in controlling tumor development and is now considered one of the hallmarks of cancer. The last few years has seen an explosion in immunotherapy as a targeted strategy to fight cancer without damaging healthy cells. In this way, long-lasting results are elicited by activation of an antitumor immune response, utilizing the body's own surveillance mechanisms to reprogram the tumour microenvironment. The next challenge is to ensure targeted delivery of these therapies for increased efficacy and reduction in immune-related adverse events. Liposomes are an attractive drug delivery system providing versatility in their formulation including material type, charge, size and importantly surface chemical modifications that confer their tumour specificity. These tunable properties make them an attractive platform for the treatment of cancer. In this chapter, we will discuss clinically approved immunotherapies and those undergoing clinical trials together with, recent liposomal approaches for enhanced specificity and efficacy.

Keywords: immunotherapy, liposomes, nanocarriers, systemic delivery, cancer

1. Introduction

Cancer cannot be considered a mass of isolated tumor cells, but instead, it relies on several interactions with the surrounding microenvironment. Indeed, in response to evolving environmental conditions and oncogenic signals from growing tumors, the tumor microenvironment (TME) continually changes during cancer progression, highlighting the need to consider its influence on metastasis as a dynamic process, and to understand how tumor cells drive the construction of their own niche [1, 2]. The TME stromal compartment comprises both nonmalignant cells such as fibroblasts, myofibroblasts, endothelial cells and immune cells as well as signaling molecules including growth factors, chemokines, cytokines, extracellular matrices

 IntechOpen

(ECMs) and matrix-degrading enzymes that act together to promote cancer progression and metastasis. Indeed, they all become educated by the tumor to acquire pro-tumorigenic functions [3]. Based on these considerations, in the last few years, several strategies to fight cancer have been developed to alter the TME and effectively reprogram it [4]. These include chemotherapy, targeted therapy, immunotherapy and combinations of these therapies. Chemotherapy elicits anti-cancer effects by acting on cancer cell survival and proliferation, but it can also affect the TME for instance by increasing anti-tumor immune cells. However, patients have poor tolerance and can develop strong drug resistance. Therefore, there is a need to reduce side effects to chemotherapy [4]. Targeted therapies for specific TME components or signaling pathways have become the key to suppressing cancer proliferation and invasion. For example, Lee et al. found that bortezomib (BTZ) and phenobarbital (PST) reduced the survival rate of cancer-associated fibroblasts (CAFs) by inducing caspase-3-mediated apoptosis, thereby inhibiting the proliferation of cancer cells in a breast cancer mouse transplantation model [5]. Another promising strategy is immunotherapy, therapeutics that utilize the body's immune system to reprogram or activate anti-tumor immunity to kill tumor cells, without damaging normal cells. For instance, it has been demonstrated that molecules usually expressed on activated T cells, such as the immune checkpoint proteins CTLA-4 and PD-1 play a crucial role in the immunosuppression observed in the TME [6]. For this reason, several monoclonal antibodies (mAbs) targeting CTLA-4, PD-1 or PD-L1 have been developed and tested in clinical trials for the treatment of several types of cancers [7–10].

However, the promise of providing long-lasting results where other therapies have failed has not yet been realized as they are faced with a number of challenges including immune-related adverse events due to low specificity in tumor cell targeting. The use of smart drug delivery systems such as liposomes could help overcome these challenges. This chapter will give an overview of the current immunotherapy landscape and the use of liposomes to directly deliver anticancer immune therapies to tumor sites.

2. Immunotherapies

Cancer immunotherapy focuses on modulation and use of the patient's own immune system or agents that activate or enhance the immune system's recognition and killing of tumor cells [3–5]. Modulating the immune system to target cancer is a successful treatment for some solid malignancies. However, some cancers are immunogenically cold [11]. This nomenclature is given to tumours that have fewer immune cells and decreased cancer antigen expression leading to an intrinsic resistance to immunotherapies. In these 'cold' malignancies, the TME acts as a cloak to mask cancer cells from host's immune system, even in the presence of novel immunotherapies (**Figure 1**). Several approaches including cell-based therapies, cytokines, oncolytic viruses and immune checkpoint inhibitors have been approved for clinical use by the Food and Drug Administration (FDA) or in clinical trials (**Table 1**).

Cell-based immunotherapies manipulate or stimulate autologous immune cells that specifically target abnormal antigens expressed on the surface of tumor cells [52]. These include lymphocytes, macrophages, dendritic cells, natural killer cells and cytotoxic T lymphocytes (**Table 1**). However, induction of nutrient depletion and activation of negative immune regulatory pathways by cancer cells contribute to an immunosuppressive TME that compromises anti-tumor immune pathways and therefore

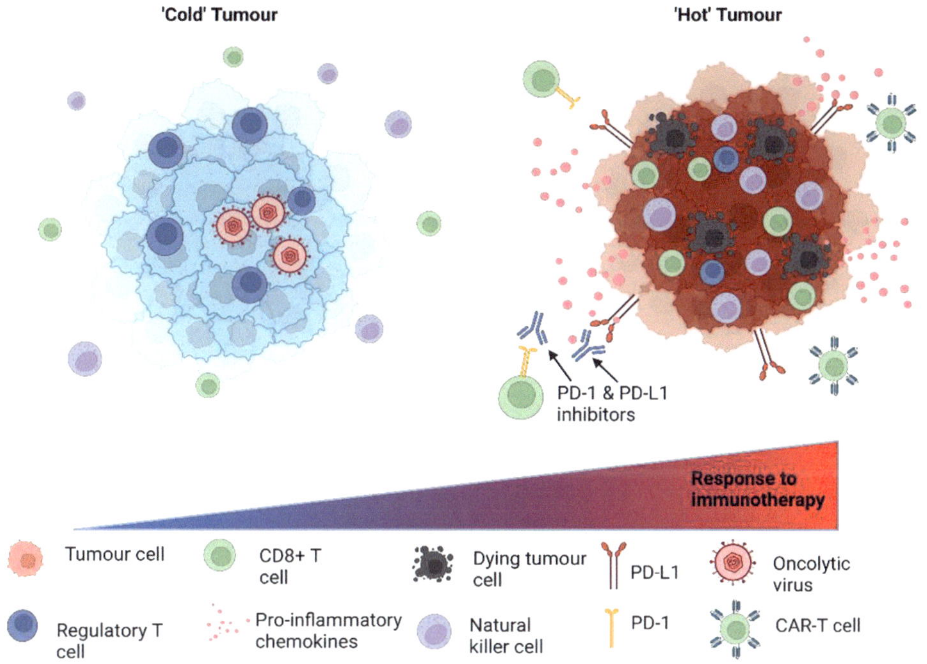

Figure 1.
Inflaming the cold tumour microenvironment using immunotherapies. 'Cold' tumors demonstrate an immunosuppressive environment with the exclusion of immune cells including Tregs, CD8+ T cells and natural killer cells from the TME resulting in poor prognosis and response to immunotherapy. 'Hot' tumor types demonstrate high immune cell infiltration and expression of pro-inflammatory markers. Immunotherapies inhibit tumor cells from deactivating T cells via PD-1, PD-L1 and CTLA-4 blockade and augment immune cell recruitment and activation via cytokine therapy to enhance tumor lysis. Created using Biorender.

the therapeutic effect of cell-based immunotherapy. This is seen in the stimulation of immunosuppressive Tregs and MDSCs [53] and patterns of expression of immune checkpoint inhibitors by activated T cells [8, 54]. Playing a crucial role in the immunosuppression observed in the TME, PD-1 and CTLA-4, through interaction with their ligands (PD-L1/PD-L2 and CD80/CD86 respectively), transmit inhibitory signals to T cells [55], thus suppressing effector T cell activation and function. Crucially, upregulation of PD-L1 and CTLA-4 on the surface of tumor cells has been detected in recent years [56] resulting in the development of mAbs targeting PD-1, PD-L1, PD-L2 and CTLA-4 for blockage of these immunosuppressive pathways [7, 8, 53–56]. Classified as immune checkpoint inhibitors, these mAbs have undergone a number of clinical trials for the treatment of several types of cancers [7–10, 12].

Manipulation of the TME by cancer cells is facilitated by cytokines and growth factors and it is well known that deregulated cytokine production and aberrant cytokine signaling can lead to altered cell growth, differentiation and apoptosis as well as the secretion of factors that foster cancer progression and immune evasion [57, 58]. Thus, cytokine therapy has been explored in the treatment of cancer to enhance anti-tumoral immunity [40, 59]. Currently three cytokines have been approved by the FDA for use in cancer patients: recombinant interleukin IL-2 (Proleukin; Chiron) and two variants of recombinant interferon alpha 2 called IFNα2a (Roferon-A; Roche) and IFNα2b (Intron-A; Merk & Co) (**Table 1**).

Oncolytic viruses (OVs), as a new therapeutic agent, offer a two-pronged attack mechanism. Their direct tumour killing is afforded in the first place by specific viral

Immunotherapy type	Drug name	Mechanism	Phase	Tumour type	References
DCs-based Vaccine	Sipuleucel-T	Patients' APCs activated by PAP and GM-CSF	Approved by FDA	Advanced prostate cancer	[12–14]
CAR-T cell therapy	Kymriah	Patient's T cells are engineered to target a protein called CD19	Approved by FDA	B-cell acute lymphoblastic leukaemia	[15, 16]
CAR-T cell therapy	Yescarta	Patient's T cells are engineered to target a protein called CD19	Approved by FDA	Large B-cell lymphoma	[17]
NK cell therapy	oNKord	NKs generated *ex vivo* from umbilical cord blood progenitor cells.	Phase I clinical trial	Acute myeloid leukaemia	[18–21]
Immune checkpoint inhibitor	Ipilimumab	Anti-CTLA-4 mAb	Approved by FDA	Unresectable or MM	[10, 22–27]
Immune checkpoint inhibitor	Nivolumab	Anti-PD-1 mAb	Approved by FDA	NSCLC, MM, HL, SCCHN, MUC	[28–31]
Immune checkpoint inhibitor	Pembrolizumab	Anti-PD-1 mAb	Approved by FDA	NSCLC, MM, HL, SCCHN, MUC	[32–35]
Immune checkpoint inhibitor	Durvalumab	Anti-PD-L1 mAb	Approved by FDA	MUC	[36]
Immune checkpoint inhibitor	Avelumab	Anti-PD-L1 mAb	Approved by FDA	Metastatic Merkel carcinoma	[37]
Immune checkpoint inhibitor	Atezolimumab	Anti-PD-L1 mAb	Approved by FDA	NSCLC, MUC	[38]
Immune checkpoint inhibitor	CA-170	Anti-PD-L1/ PD-L2 and VISTA mAb	Phase I clinical trial	Lymphomas and solid cancers	[10, 39]
Cytokine	Proleukin	IL-2	Approved by FDA	Metastatic melanoma, RCC	[40, 41]
Cytokine	Roferon-A	IFN-α2a	Approved by FDA	HCL, CML	[40, 41]

Immunotherapy type	Drug name	Mechanism	Phase	Tumour type	References
Cytokine	Intron-A	IFN-α2b	Approved by FDA	AIDS-related Kaposi's sarcoma, melanoma, FL, multiple myeloma, HCL, CIN	[40, 41]
Oncolytic virus	T-Vec (Herpes simplex virus)	Cancer cells killing and GM-CSF expression for APCs recruitment	Approved by FDA	Advanced melanoma	[42–44]
Oncolytic virus	JX-594 (Vaccinia virus)	Cancer cells killing and GM-CSF expression	Phase I clinical trail	Melanoma, HCC	[45, 46]
Oncolytic virus	CG0070 (Adenovirus)	Cancer cells killing (viral replication under the control of Rb)	Phase I clinical trail	Non-muscle invasive urothelial cancer	[47–49]
Oncolytic virus	Reolysin (Reovirus)	Cancer cells killing (viral replication under the control of Ras)	Approved by FDA	Malignant glioma, metastatic breast cancer	[50, 51]

Table 1.
Main immunotherapeutic agents approved by the FDA or in clinical trials for cancer treatment.

replication within cancer cells resulting in oncolysis. This provides self-amplification and release of viral progeny for infection of neighbouring tumour cells. Oncolysis also releases tumor antigens and following uptake by antigen presenting cells (APC), indirectly induces a systemic anti-tumor immunity through both innate and adaptive immune pathways [42, 43, 60, 61].

As therapeutic agents they also offer versatility via genetic modification to maximise their features. They can be engineered to increase tropism towards specific cancers via capsid insertion of ligands for enhanced tumor cell binding [43, 62, 63]. Additional transgenes can be inserted for expression of proteins designed to further amplify immune activation at the tumor site. Moreover, strategies to improve selective replication in cancer cells and hence their safety, include the deletion/insertion of tissue- or cell type- specific promoters to induce gene expression in tumor cells [64]; or the placement of viral genes under the control of tissue specific elements. Despite these attractive properties, successful use of OVs in the clinic to date, have been limited to direct tumor injection as systemic delivery results in rapid clearance whilst in circulation, thus preventing tumor targeting. For these to be used more widely in the clinic, strategies are needed to protect the virus in the blood stream so that tumors in inaccessible locations can be treated [65]. Whilst in the last decade immunotherapy has become a viable treatment option for some cancers, for many patients this is still limited due to its low response rates as a monotherapy [66].

Combination therapy is instead a treatment modality that combines two or more therapeutic agents to fight cancer. It is probably the most effective approach because it targets key pathways in a characteristically synergistic or an additive manner, reducing drug resistance and providing therapeutic anti-cancer benefits, such as reducing tumor growth and metastatic potential, arresting mitotically active cells, reducing cancer stem cell populations, and inducing apoptosis [67]. However, obtaining these achievements is complicated and an easier and more promising approach could be the use of nanotechnology. Indeed, the use of nanomedicine has several advantages such as the early diagnosis of disease and the combination of different therapeutic agents for overcoming cancer resistance [68]. Moreover, nanoparticles can be fabricated with unique characteristics including their material type, size, shape, charge and surface chemical modifications for tunable optimization [69]. Indeed, changing nanoparticles physical and chemical properties has an important effect on their kinetics of internalization, biodistribution, cellular uptake, immunogenicity and loading efficiency [70, 71] making them the most promising platform for biomedical applications [69].

3. Liposomes

Traditionally known as liposomes, lipopolymers, solid lipid nanoparticles, nanostructured lipid nanoparticles, microemulsions and nanoemulsions, lipid nanoparticles are used primarily for the release of small molecules, peptides, genes and monoclonal antibodies [72]. Liposomes consist of spherical vesicles having one or more lipid layers containing an aqueous core. The structure of a conventional liposome allows the encapsulation of both hydrophilic and lipophilic agents in the lipid layers or in the internal compartment, respectively (**Figure 2**) [73, 74]. Depending on the water solubility of the payload, they can be encapsulated in the aqueous core (hydrophilic drugs) or in surrounding bilayer of the liposome (hydrophobic drugs) [75]. They are physically stable, and unlike other nanoparticles, they are not covalently bound. As a delivery system, LNPs offer many advantages, including simplicity of simulation, self-assembly, biocompatibility, high bioavailability, the ability to carry large payloads, and a range of physicochemical properties that can control their biological properties [76]. Lipid nanoparticles are the most common class of FDA-approved nanomedicine drugs (**Table 1**). Among them, the liposome-encapsulated form of Doxorubicin (Doxil) approved by the FDA in 1995 for the treatment of ovarian cancer and AIDS-related Kaposi's sarcoma can be considered the first success in this field [73, 74, 77, 78].

Other examples that need to be mentioned are liposomal daunorubicin (DaunoXome) for treatment of poor-risk acute leukemia [79], Liposome-encapsulated doxorubicin citrate (Myocet) for breast cancer therapy [80], the Liposomal cytarabine (DepoCyte) for the treatment of neoplastic meningitis [81], the vincristine sulfate liposome injection (Marqibo) for childhood and adult hematologic malignancies [82] and the irinotecan liposome injection (Nivyde) for the treatment of metastatic pancreatic cancer [83]. There are approximately 1862 clinical trials involving the use of liposomes in cancer therapy [84]. These liposomal formulations of chemotherapies were designed to overcome problems with severe side effects (nausea, fatigue, diarrhea, hair loss, disruption of mouth, pharynx mucosa, and bone marrow [85, 86]) as well as improvements in both the drug bioavailability at the tumor site

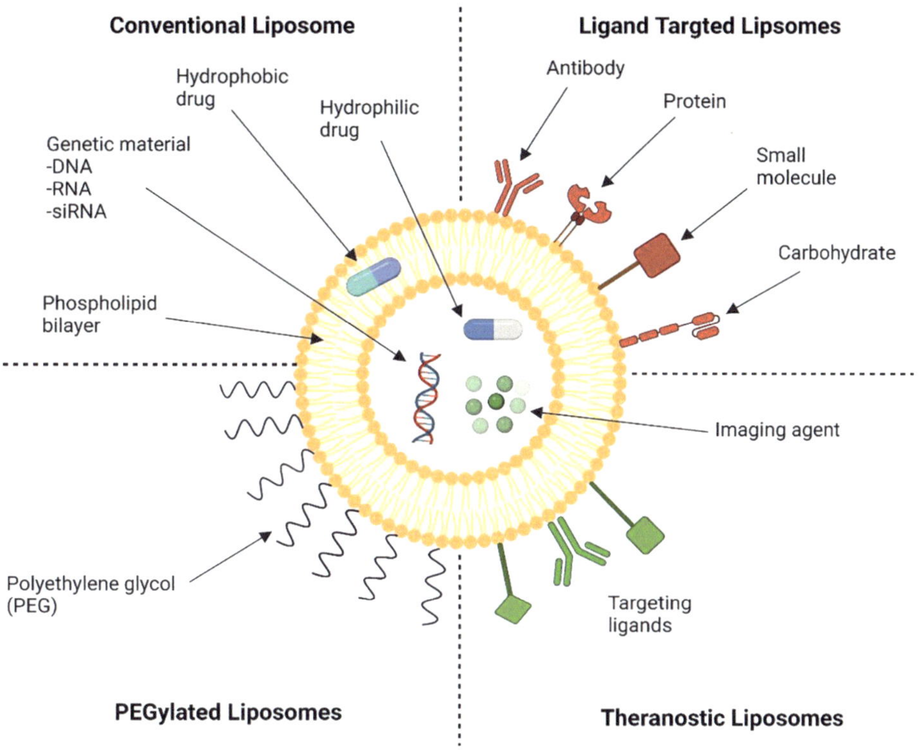

Figure 2.
Schematic of liposomes comprising outer phospholipid layer. PEGylated liposomes contain a layer of polyethylene glycol (PEG) on the surface of liposomes. Targeted liposomes contain a specific targeting ligand to target a cancer site. Multifunctional theranostic liposomes can be used for diagnosis and treatment of solid tumors.

and its pharmacokinetic properties in order to deliver the active drug molecules to the site of action, without affecting healthy cells.

3.1 Liposomes and chemotherapy

The mechanism of action of Doxil is based on the use of sterically stabilized (composed of high Tm phospholipids and cholesterol), PEGylated nano-liposomes to prolong drug circulation time and allow efficicent extravasation via the EPR effect. Additionally, stable loading of doxorubicin (DOX) as well as DOX release at the tumor target is provided by a transmembrane ammonium sulfate gradient [78]. Unlike Doxil, the Myocet liposome does not have a PEG coating, but it seems to have less cardiotoxicity. It is approved in the European Union and in Canada for the treatment of metastatic breast cancer in combination with cyclophosphamide, but it has not been approved by the FDA for use in the United States [87].

Another anthracycline to utilize the advantages of liposomal packaging is daunorubicin. DaunoXome contaisn an aqueous solution of the citrate salt of daunorubicin encapsulated within lipid vesicles composed of a lipid bilayer of distearoylphosphatidylcholine and cholesterol [88]. By protecting the entrapped compound from chemical and enzymatic degradation, DaunoXome increases its biocompatibility and bioavailability by reducing uptake by normal tissues and minimizing protein binding respectively. It is FDA approved to treat AIDS related Kaposi's sarcoma. It is also commonly used to treat specific types of leukemia and non-Hodgkin lymphoma [88].

Another example of lipid-nanocarrier for chemotherapeutic agents is Depocyte, a liposomal formulation of cytosine arabinoside (Ara-C) which is a cytosine analog with arabinose sugar that kills cancer cells by interfering with DNA synthesis [89]. Ara-C has a short plasma half-life, low lipophilicity, stability and limited bioavailability. DepoCyte consists of multivesicular lipid-based polymeric liposomal carriers composed of cholesterol, glycerol trioleate, triglyceride, phospholipids that increase the Ara-C half-life and consequently in the treatment of lymphomatous meningitis [90].

Vincristine (VCR) is a vinca alkaloid that is thought to work by interfering with cancer cell growth during mitosis and it used for treatment of hematologic malignancies and solid tumors. Its main challenge is that it has a diffuse distribution and tissue binding that can limit drug efficacy and generate several side effects [82]. To overcome this, VCR has been encapsulated in sphingomyelin/cholesterol liposomes to produce a vinCRIStine sulfate liposome injection called Marqibo [82]. It is specifically indicated for the treatment of adults with Philadelphia chromosome-negative (Ph-) acute lymphoblastic leukemia in second or greater relapse or whose disease has progressed following two or more anti-leukemia therapies.

The topoisomerase I inhibitor Irinotecan is another example of how lipid carriers can increase chemotherapy efficacy and reduce toxicity. Irinotecan is indeed a drug currently used in the treatment of multiple solid tumors, such as metastatic colorectal cancer (mCRC), small-cell lung cancer, non-small-cell lung cancer, gastric cancer, and cervical cancer [91]. The main challenges in irinotecan usage are the acute toxicities caused by it and its fast elimination that can strongly limit its clinical applications [92, 93]. For this reason, the liposomal formulation Onivyde has been developed to improve the pharmacokinetics and reducing host toxicity. Onivyde was approved by the US Food and Drug Administration (FDA) in October 2015 as a combination regimen for patients with gemcitabine-based chemotherapy-resistant metastatic pancreatic cancer [91].

Considering all these advancements, it is clear that liposomes have overcome the limitations of conventional chemotherapy by improving drug bioavailability and stability and minimizing their side effects by site-specific targeted delivery. This success has paved the way for the use of liposomal agents in the field of cancer immunotherapy together with additional modifications of the liposomal surface, facilitating their active targeting to tumors. Whilst passive targeting relies on the EPR effect for accumulation of liposomes within tumors, active targeting is obtained by linking to liposomes membrane specific ligands that bind specific antigens on cancer cells [75] (**Figure 2**). Next, we describe these modifications in the context of liposomal delivery of immunotherapeutics.

3.2 Liposomal immunotherapies

Improving CAR-T cell therapy against solid tumors has recently adopted the use of lipid nanoparticles in order to address the issues surrounding the presence of an immunosuppressive TME that can decrease the treatment efficacy [71]. A recent study by Zhang and colleagues showed promising results in a model of murine breast cancer to overcome this obstacle using infusions of lipid nanoparticles coated with the tumor-targeting peptide iRGD and loaded with a combination of a PI3K inhibitor to block immunosuppressive tumor cells activity and α-GalCer (an iNKT cell activator). The investigators demonstrated a switch in the TME from immunosuppressive to stimulatory thereby enabling tumor-specific CAR-T cells to home to the tumor, undergo robust expansion and trigger tumor regression [94] during a 2 week therapeutic window. This strategy has been applied to a number of immunotherapies (**Table 2**) to assist in their delivery, efficacy and safety as follows.

3.2.1 Liposomes and ICI's

The development of immune checkpoint inhibitors (ICIs) has been a major breakthrough in cancer immunotherapy. However, only a small percentage of patients exhibit durable responses under monotherapy and their increasing use has led to the discovery of immune-related adverse events (irAEs) including myopathy [112], immune-related myasthenia gravis (irMG) [113] and pneumonitis [114] to name a few. Whilst BMS-202 (a small molecule inhibitor of PD-1/PD-L1) loaded liposomes have inhibited tumor growth in a model of triple negative breast cancer (TNBC) [115] and pancreatic cancer when combined with photothermal therapy [96], there is now a trend towards combination therapy (**Table 2**). For example, amplification of the therapeutic potential of DOX-loaded biomimetic hybrid nanovesicles (DOX@LINV) (synthesized by fusing artificial liposomes with tumor-derived nanovesicles, facilitating both targeted delivery of DOX to tumor tissue and eliciting effective immunogenic cell death response to improve the immunogenicity of the tumor) by combination treatment with aPD-1 antibody prolonged survival of B16F10 tumor-bearing mice by 33% [116]. Additionally, the utilization of PD1/PD-L1 mAbs as surface ligands for enhanced tumor targeting of nanoparticles is an emerging strategy whereby PD-L1 targeted DOX [117] and catalase [118] immunoliposomes are promising candidates for melanoma immunotherapy.

3.2.2 Liposomes and antibodies

One of the most notorious targets for interventional antibody therapy is the Human Epidermal growth factor Receptor 2 (HER2) which is involved in important stages of growth and cell differentiation and is overexpressed by HER2 positive breast cancer cells. Targeting HER2 positive cancers can be achieved by coating liposomes with an anti-HER2 monoclonal antibody [119] and in recent years, several targeted therapy options for HER2-positive breast cancer has been developed including Pertuzumab (Perjeta), Trastuzumab (Herceptin), Tucatinib (Tukysa), Neratinib (Nerlynx), Margetuximab (Margenza), DS-8201 (Enhertu), and Ado-trastuzumab emtansine or T-DM1 (Kadcyla) [120]. In particular, Herceptin was FDA approved in 1998 for the treatment of HER2-positive breast cancers [121] and has been studied extensively since including using various nano delivery systems. For example, Elamir et al., functionalized calcein and Doxorubicin-loaded pegylated liposomes with Herceptin and utilized Low-Frequency ultrasound for their controlled release to enhance uptake by cancer cells in vitro, paving the way for in vivo studies [119].

Anchoring antibodies to the surface of liposomes to enable targeted delivery (**Figure 1**) can also be performed within the circulation. For instance, in 2004 van Broekhoven et al. targeted DCs through anti-DEC-205 or anti-CD11c mAbs located on the surface of liposomes containing tumor antigens (B16 melanoma antigens or lipopolysaccharide), thus inducing potent anti-tumor immunity both in vitro and in vivo [122, 123].

Another molecule overexpressed by cancer cells is the vascular endothelial growth factor (VEGF) that increases angiogenesis for enhanced tumor growth. Indeed, it binds two VEGF receptors (VEGF receptor-1 and VEGF receptor-2) on vascular

Immunotherapy type	Delivery platform	Tumour type	Reference
Immune checkpoint inhibitors			
PD-L1	Cerasome nanoparticle loaded with Paclitaxel and decorated with PD-L1	Breast, colon	[95]
BMS-202 (PD-1/PD-L1 inhibitor)	BMS-202 loaded thermosensitive liposomes	Pancreatic	[96]
Monoclonal antibodies			
Intravenous immunoglobulin	PEGylated nanoliposome encapsulating the antibody	Colorectal	[97]
Anti-EGFR antibody	Porphyrin containing liposomal cersaome decorated with Cetuximab	Colorectal carcinoma	[98]
HER2	HER2 targeted PEGylated liposome	Metastatic breast cancer	[99]
Oncolytic viruses			
Oncolytic Adenovirus	Liposome-cloaked oncolytic adenovirus conjugated to tumour homing E.coli	Lung	[100]
Oncolytic Adenovirus	CCL2-coated liposomes for monocytic cell delivery	Prostate	[101]
Cancer vaccines			
Epitope vaccine	Mannose decorated liposomes activate DC maturation for enhanced cytotoxic T lymphocyte response	Metastatic breast cancer	[102]
LAG3-Ig + P5 tumour antigen	PEGylated liposome bearing surface conjugated LAG3-Ig and P5 tumour antigen	Breast	[103]
Synthetic long peptides	Liposome loaded with tumour specific synthetic long peptides	Lung, melanoma	[104]
Combination treatments			
Tumour vaccine of antigen epitopes + IDO inhibitor	Lipid hybrid nanovesicle-based liposomes containing tumour vaccine and immune checkpoint inhibitor	Melanoma	[105]
Anti-PD-L1 + Docetaxel	Liposome co-loaded with PD-L1 antibody and Docetaxel	Melanoma	[106]
siRNA-PD-L1 + Imatinib	Liposomal co-delivery of siRNA-PD-L1 and Imatinib	Melanoma	[107]
Interleukin-2 (IL-2) + anti-PD-L1 + Imiquimod	C25 antibody modified liposomes containing a combination of treatments attached to the surface of T regulatory cell	Melanoma	[108]
Other immune system modulators			
Interferon-gamma (IFN-γ)	PEGylated liposomes containing IFN-γ	Colon	[109]

Immunotherapy type	Delivery platform	Tumour type	Reference
Small immunostimulatory RNA	Liposomes containing immunostimulatory RNA	Melanoma	[110]
Interleukin-15 (IL-15)	Folate receptor targeted liposome containing IL-15 plasmid	Colon	[111]

Table 2.
Preclinical models of liposomal immunotherapeutics in development.

endothelial cells allowing tumor vasculature to grow exponentially thereby promoting cancer progression and metastasis [124]. Several agents, including antibodies and soluble receptor constructs, have been developed to target the VEGF system. The drug that is currently most widely used in the clinical practice to modulate VEGF-A is the humanized monoclonal antibody Bevacizumab, approved by the FDA and EMA for the treatment of metastatic colorectal cancer, non-small cell lung cancer, breast cancer and glioblastoma multiforme in combination with chemotherapy (**Table 1**) [125]. Several studies have been also conducted to improve bevacizumab efficacy and reduce its toxicity by using lipid nanocarriers. For instance, Kuesters and Campbell demonstrated that cationic pegylated liposomes that preferentially target the tumor vasculature, can be conjugated with bevacizumab and can increase its cellular uptake and tumor targeting in vitro [126]. Moreover, bevacizumab is extensively studied for ovarian cancer treatment since the combination of surgery and platinum-based chemotherapy is initially very effective in treating this cancer, but most patients will experience a recurrence because they acquire platinum resistance. To overcome these challenges, a phase II clinical trial (NCT04753216) is studying the combination of irinotecan liposome and bevacizumab in women with recurrent, platinum resistant ovarian cancer and the predicted results are that the liposomal encapsulation will enhance drug delivery and bioavailability, thereby improving efficacy and reducing toxicity [127]. These examples mentioned above, strengthen the idea that the use of therapy combination together with nanoparticles, in particular liposomes, as delivery systems, could strongly increase the cancer treatments efficacy, also overcoming drug resistance experienced by patients, and reduce their associated toxicities.

3.2.3 Liposomes and oncolytic viruses

The encapsulation of OVs inside lipid nanoparticles is another strategy that has demonstrated encouraging results in the last few years (**Table 2**). Acting as a protective shield, the phospholipid coating can hide viral epitopes thus reducing OV neutralization by pre-existing Abs upon systemic administration as seen by Chen et al. [128]. Not only that, but the efficacy of this encapsulated ZD55-IL-24 oncolytic adenovirus was demonstrated via inhibition of HCC proliferation and an enhanced anti-tumor immune response in vivo. Similarly, a separate study involvingliposome-encapsulated plasmid DNA of telomerase specific oncolytic adenovirus (TelomeScan) also recorded shielding from adenovirus-neutralizing Abs following intravenous administration into immune-competent mice compared to the naked virus together with potent anti-tumor effects on colon carcinoma cells both in vitro and in vivo [101, 129]. Shielding the viral epitopes from immunosurveillance has not only reduced their rapid clearance from the circulation but the addition of targeting ligands on the surface increases their accumulation at target sites and reduces off-target side effects. Successful encapsulation of AD[I/PPT-E1A] into CCL2-coated liposomes were preferentially taken up by CCR2-expressing monocytes within the circulation thereby exploiting the recruitment of circulating monocytes by tumors for their targeted delivery [101]. This resulted in a significant reduction in tumor size and pulmonary metastases in pre-clinical model of prostate cancer at a viral titer 3 logs lower than AD[I/PPT-E1A] alone. Taken together, liposome-assisted delivery cannot only target OVs via the circulation to inaccessible tumors but reduction in concentration of virus required for efficacy provides additional safety and cost benefits.

3.2.4 Liposomes and immune-gene therapy

Liposomes have been studied in the field of cancer gene therapy for the targeting of genes involved in the development of cancer (**Table 2**). For example, the liposomal delivery of a stimulator of interferon genes (STING) agonist has augmented cytokine therapy. In a model of metastatic melanoma, investigators saw an increase in IFNγ production by tumor-associated APCs, leading to anti-tumor immunity enhancement and cancer regression compared to the free drug [130]. Further advancements in lipid nanotechnology for the delivery of gene therapy have developed strategies for controlled release, improved therapeutic loading and faster route to market as follows.

With their positive charge, cationic liposomes, can be used to easily encapsulate plasmid DNA (pDNA), messenger RNA (mRNA), or small interfering RNA (siRNA) via electrostatic interactions [131]. An important example is the T7 peptide modified core-shell nanoparticles (named as T7-LPC/siRNA NPs). The core-shell structure of T7-LPC/siRNA NPs enables them to encapsulate siRNA in the core and protect it from RNase degradation during circulation. Both in vitro and in vivo results show that this system can efficiently deliver the EGFR siRNA into breast cancer cells through receptor mediated endocytosis and down-regulate the EGFR expression [132]. Furthermore, plasmids can be encapsulated in lipid nanocarriers whereby a tumor-targeted liposomal nano delivery complex (SGT-94) carrying a plasmid encoding RB94, a truncated form of the RB gene, has shown promising results in metastatic genitourinary cancer in terms of selective tumor targeting and tolerability [133].

The first marketed RNA drug, Onpattro®, was launched by Alnylam Pharmaceuticals in 2018. Onpattro® comprises lipid nanoparticles (LNPs) prepared from ionizable lipids for siRNA encapsulation and delivery [134]. LNPs have since become the preferential vector for nucleic acid delivery. LNPs are constructed using phospholipids with ionizable lipids and other supporting phospholipids to complete the particle [76, 135]. A high degree of encapsulation is achieved by mutual adsorption of the nucleic acid's negative charge and the ionizable lipid's positive charge. When LNPs enter the body, the cytolysis mechanism mediated by low-density lipoproteins allows the nanoparticles to be successfully taken up by cells [136]. The endosome successfully releases the phagocytosed LNPs and transports them to the cytoplasm for expression, producing the corresponding protein.

These mRNA vaccines have gained a lot of attention due to their good safety profiles, successful preventative effects and rapid development of mRNA technology, making them very competitive [137]. Indeed, thanks to the prior optimization of mRNA and extensive basic research and testing of lipid nanoparticles, the mRNA vaccine against SARS-CoV-2 took less than a year from the publication of the virus sequence to the launch of the vaccine, and demonstrated an efficacy rate of over 90% [138]. This was previously unimaginable and unattainable. Application of this technology for further optimization and improvement to CAR-T therapy has utilized lipid nanoparticles as a medium to target mRNA delivery to T cells and constructed CAR- T directly *in vivo* to treat heart failure symptoms in mice [139]. Upon delivery of mRNA to mice, large mRNA molecules are captured by T cells, allowing T cells to gain the ability to target cardiac fibroblasts specifically. The mRNA successfully encoded T cells in mice with heart failure, resulting in a significant reduction in myocardial fibrosis and heart repair to near normal size and function. The in vivo construction of CAR-T was accomplished through mRNA targeted delivery, and mRNA-LNP-targeted delivery is far less costly than traditional cellular therapies [140].

Other non-viral vectors for gene transfer into tumor cells is the use of lipoplexes (LPX) and micelleplexes and are proving promising in phase I/II clinical trials for advanced melanoma treatment. By protecting its' RNA payload from extracellular ribonucleases, these vectors improve cell uptake and hence gene expression. For example, in a B16-F10 murine melanoma tumor model, a micelleplex made of an acid-activatable cationic micelle, a photosensitizer and a small interfering RNA (siRNA) was able to inhibit PD-L1 resulting in inhibition of both primary tumour growth and formation of distant metastases formation compared to photothermal therapy alone [141]. This was achieved through its activatable composition, only switching "on" upon internalization in the acidic endocytic vesicles of tumor cells, demonstrating the versatility of these particles.

4. Route to clinic/challenges

Although nanoparticle drug delivery technology has now been extensively researched, the prevalence of nanomedicines is far below expectations [9, 56]. One of the main challenges is that the current processes used for liposome manufacturing suffers from many severe problems such as high costs of production related to multi-step batch processes, the need to use specialized tools and equipment for particle size reduction and limited batch sizes [77].

Polymeric materials were the most common delivery vehicles used by early scientists, such as polyethyleneimine (PEI), polyamine ester (PBAE), chitosan, etc. [142]. However, the application of polymeric materials has stalled at the pre-clinical trial stage [143]. In a study investigating PEI delivery of DNA to the lungs, the poor breakdown of PEI raised concerns regarding accumulation of the polymer as well as specific side effects, particularly for repeated treatment administration [144]. Most polymeric materials used for nucleic acid delivery require modification of fatty acid chains to improve their safety. A team of researchers developed a branched polyamine polymer for mRNA encapsulation and prepared polymeric RNA nanoparticles whereby these vaccine recipients successfully expressed antibodies against Zika and Ebola viruses [145]. Although LNPs have been used on a large scale (in particular how to achieve higher therapeutic efficacy as discussed) optimization of the production process is also required for successful translation of these formulations to the clinic. This includes optimization of the LNP production process, control of the LNP characteristics, shelf-life, regulatory considerations and cost effectiveness.

5. Conclusions

The possibility that immunotherapy could replace surgery and other forms of cancer treatment is being entertained for the first time. However, this is not all good news as many of these immunotherapies are associated with potentially serious side effects, linked to inflammation in the bowel, lung, heart, skin and other organs. Liposomes display superiority as a delivery platform for cancer immunotherapy with the potential to overcome many of the challenges related to their systemic delivery and toxicity. However, for this to become reality, the less than satisfactory targeting efficiency of liposomes needs to be addressed to achieve improved clinical performance.

Acknowledgements

Financial support provided by Cancer Research UK (CRUK grant reference: C25574/A24321) and the European Union's Horizon 2020 research and innovation programme under the Marie Sklodowska Curie grant (agreement No 777682 CANCER).

Conflict of interest

The authors declare no conflict of interest.

Author details

Alessandra Iscaro†, Faith H.N. Howard†, Zidi Yang, Fern Jenkins and Munitta Muthana*
University of Sheffield, Sheffield, UK

*Address all correspondence to: m.muthana@sheffield.ac.uk

† Joint first authors.

References

[1] Hanahan D, Coussens LM. Accessories to the crime: Functions of cells recruited to the tumor microenvironment. Cancer Cell. 2012;**21**(3):309-322

[2] Hanahan D, Weinberg RA. Hallmarks of cancer: The next generation. Cell. 2011;**144**(5):646-674

[3] Josson S et al. Tumor-stromal interactions influence radiation sensitivity in epithelial- versus mesenchymal-like prostate cancer cells. Journal of Oncology. 2010;**2010**:10

[4] Li H et al. Underlying mechanisms and drug intervention strategies for the tumour microenvironment. Journal of Experimental & Clinical Cancer Research. 2021;**40**(1):97

[5] Lee HM et al. Drug repurposing screening identifies bortezomib and panobinostat as drugs targeting cancer associated fibroblasts (CAFs) by synergistic induction of apoptosis. Investigational New Drugs. 2018;**36**(4):545-560

[6] Seidel JA, Otsuka A, Kabashima K. Anti-PD-1 and anti-CTLA-4 therapies in cancer: Mechanisms of action, efficacy, and limitations. Frontiers in Oncology. 2018;**8**:86

[7] Wang Z et al. Nanoscale delivery systems for cancer immunotherapy. Materials Horizons. 2018;**5**(3):344-362

[8] Ludin A, Zon LI. Cancer immunotherapy: The dark side of PD-1 receptor inhibition. Nature. 2017;**552**(7683):41-42

[9] Alsaab HO et al. PD-1 and PD-L1 checkpoint signaling inhibition for cancer immunotherapy: Mechanism, combinations, and clinical outcome. Frontiers in Pharmacology. 2017;**8**:561

[10] Vanpouille-Box C et al. Trial watch: Immune checkpoint blockers for cancer therapy. Oncoimmunology. 2017;**6**(11):e1373237

[11] Sharma P, Allison JP. The future of immune checkpoint therapy. Science. 2015;**348**(6230):56-61

[12] Garg NK et al. RNA pulsed dendritic cells: An approach for cancer immunotherapy. Vaccine. 2013;**31**(8):1141-1156

[13] Approval Letter—Provenge. 2010. Available from: https://www.fda.gov/vaccines-blood-biologics/cellular-gene-therapy-products/provenge-sipuleucel-t

[14] L, R. U.S. FDA OKs Dendreon's Prostate Cancer Vaccine. 2010. Available from: https://www.reuters.com/article/dendreon-prostate-cancer-idUKN2919838820100429

[15] D'Aloia MM et al. CAR-T cells: The long and winding road to solid tumors. Cell Death & Disease. 2018;**9**(3):282

[16] Approval Letter—Kymriah. 2017. Available from: https://www.fda.gov/vaccines-blood-biologics/cellular-gene-therapy-products/kymriah-tisagenlecleucel

[17] Approval Letter—Yescarta. 2017. Available from: https://www.fda.gov/vaccines-blood-biologics/cellular-gene-therapy-products/yescarta-axicabtagene-ciloleucel

[18] Hofer E, Koehl U. Natural killer cell-based cancer immunotherapies:

From immune evasion to promising targeted cellular therapies. Frontiers in Immunology. 2017;**8**:745

[19] Granzin M et al. Fully automated expansion and activation of clinical-grade natural killer cells for adoptive immunotherapy. Cytotherapy. 2015;**17**(5):621-632

[20] Granzin M et al. Highly efficient IL-21 and feeder cell-driven ex vivo expansion of human NK cells with therapeutic activity in a xenograft mouse model of melanoma. Oncoimmunology. 2016;**5**(9):e1219007

[21] Spanholtz J et al. Clinical-grade generation of active NK cells from cord blood hematopoietic progenitor cells for immunotherapy using a closed-system culture process. PLoS One. 2011;**6**(6):e20740

[22] Nelson AL, Dhimolea E, Reichert JM. Development trends for human monoclonal antibody therapeutics. Nature Reviews. Drug Discovery. 2010;**9**(10):767-774

[23] Hodi FS et al. Improved survival with ipilimumab in patients with metastatic melanoma. The New England Journal of Medicine. 2010;**363**(8):711-723

[24] Buqué A et al. Trial watch: Immunomodulatory monoclonal antibodies for oncological indications. Oncoimmunology. 2015;**4**(4):e1008814

[25] Galluzzi L, Eggermont A, Kroemer G. Doubling the blockade for melanoma immunotherapy. Oncoimmunology. 2016;**5**(1):e1106127

[26] Ascierto PA, Marincola FM, Ribas A. Anti-CTLA4 monoclonal antibodies: The past and the future in clinical application. Journal of Translational Medicine. 2011;**9**:196

[27] Approval Letter—Ipilimumab. 2011. Available from: https://www.accessdata.fda.gov/drugsatfda_docs/appletter/2011/125377s000ltr.pdf#:~:text=We%20have%20approved%20your%20BLA%20for%20ipilimumab%20effective,for%20the%20treatment%20of%20unresectable%20or%20metastatic%20melanoma

[28] Weber JS et al. Nivolumab versus chemotherapy in patients with advanced melanoma who progressed after anti-CTLA-4 treatment (CheckMate 037): A randomised, controlled, open-label, phase 3 trial. The Lancet Oncology. 2015;**16**(4):375-384

[29] Borghaei H et al. Nivolumab versus docetaxel in advanced nonsquamous non-small-cell lung cancer. The New England Journal of Medicine. 2015;**373**(17):1627-1639

[30] Younes A et al. Nivolumab for classical Hodgkin's lymphoma after failure of both autologous stem-cell transplantation and brentuximab vedotin: A multicentre, multicohort, single-arm phase 2 trial. The Lancet Oncology. 2016;**17**(9):1283-1294

[31] Sharma P et al. Nivolumab in metastatic urothelial carcinoma after platinum therapy (CheckMate 275): A multicentre, single-arm, phase 2 trial. The Lancet Oncology. 2017;**18**(3):312-322

[32] Robert C et al. Anti-programmed-death-receptor-1 treatment with pembrolizumab in ipilimumab-refractory advanced melanoma: A randomised dose-comparison cohort of a phase 1 trial. Lancet. 2014;**384**(9948):1109-1117

[33] Langer CJ et al. Carboplatin and pemetrexed with or without pembrolizumab for advanced, non-squamous non-small-cell lung cancer:

A randomised, phase 2 cohort of the open-label KEYNOTE-021 study. The Lancet Oncology. 2016;**17**(11):1497-1508

[34] Chen R et al. Phase II study of the efficacy and safety of Pembrolizumab for relapsed/refractory classic Hodgkin lymphoma. Journal of Clinical Oncology. 2017;**35**(19):2125-2132

[35] Bellmunt J et al. Pembrolizumab as second-line therapy for advanced urothelial carcinoma. The New England Journal of Medicine. 2017;**376**(11):1015-1026

[36] Massard C et al. Safety and efficacy of Durvalumab (MEDI4736), an anti-programmed cell death Ligand-1 immune checkpoint inhibitor, in patients with advanced urothelial bladder cancer. Journal of Clinical Oncology. 2016;**34**(26):3119-3125

[37] Kaufman HL et al. Avelumab in patients with chemotherapy-refractory metastatic Merkel cell carcinoma: A multicentre, single-group, open-label, phase 2 trial. The Lancet Oncology. 2016;**17**(10):1374-1385

[38] Balar AV et al. Atezolizumab as first-line treatment in cisplatin-ineligible patients with locally advanced and metastatic urothelial carcinoma: A single-arm, multicentre, phase 2 trial. Lancet. 2017;**389**(10064):67-76

[39] Lazorchak AS, Patterson T, Ding Y, Sasikumar PG, Sudarshan NS, Gowda NM, et al. CA-170, an oral small molecule PD-L1 and VISTA immune checkpoint antagonist, promotes T cell immune activation and inhibits tumor growth in pre-clinical models of cancer. [abstract]. In: Proceedings of the AACR Special Conference on Tumor Immunology and Immunotherapy; 2016 Oct 20-23; Boston, MA. Philadelphia (PA): AACR, Cancer Immunol Res. 2017;**5**(3 Suppl):Abstract nr A36

[40] Waldmann TA. Cytokines in cancer immunotherapy. Cold Spring Harbor Perspectives in Biology. 2018;**10**(12):1-23

[41] García-Martínez E et al. Trial watch: Immunostimulation with recombinant cytokines for cancer therapy. OncoImmunology. 2018;**7**:16

[42] Papaioannou NE et al. Harnessing the immune system to improve cancer therapy. Annals of Translational Medicine. 2016;**4**(14):261

[43] Bommareddy PK, Shettigar M, Kaufman HL. Integrating oncolytic viruses in combination cancer immunotherapy. Nature Reviews. Immunology. 2018;**18**(8):498-513

[44] Schenk E et al. Clinical adenoviral gene therapy for prostate cancer. Human Gene Therapy. 2010;**21**(7):807-813

[45] Mastrangelo MJ et al. Intratumoral recombinant GM-CSF-encoding virus as gene therapy in patients with cutaneous melanoma. Cancer Gene Therapy. 1999;**6**(5):409-422

[46] Park BH et al. Use of a targeted oncolytic poxvirus, JX-594, in patients with refractory primary or metastatic liver cancer: A phase I trial. The Lancet Oncology. 2008;**9**(6):533-542

[47] Ramesh N et al. CG0070, a conditionally replicating granulocyte macrophage colony-stimulating factor—Armed oncolytic adenovirus for the treatment of bladder cancer. Clinical Cancer Research. 2006;**12**(1):305-313

[48] Burke JM et al. A first in human phase 1 study of CG0070, a GM-CSF expressing oncolytic adenovirus, for the treatment of nonmuscle invasive bladder cancer. The Journal of Urology. 2012;**188**(6):2391-2397

[49] Fountzilas C, Patel S, Mahalingam D. Review: Oncolytic virotherapy, updates and future directions. Oncotarget. 2017;**8**(60):102617-102639

[50] Oncolytics Biotech Inc. Announces Receipt of FDA Orphan Drug Designation for REOLYSIN. 2015. Available from: https://www.prnewswire.com/news-releases/oncolytics-biotech-inc-announces-receipt-of-orphan-drug-designation-from-the-us-fda-for-malignant-gliomas-500265141.html#:~:text=CALGARY%2C%20April%2017%2C%202015%20%2FPRNewswire%2F%20-%20Oncolytics%20Biotech,REOLYSIN%20%C2%AE%2C%20for%20the%20treatment%20of%20malignant%20glioma

[51] Oncolytics Biotech Inc. Announces FDA Fast Track Designation for REOLYSIN in Metastatic Breast Cancer. 2017. Available from: https://www.americanpharmaceuticalreview.com/1315-News/337402-Oncolytics-Biotech-Announces-FDA-Fast-Track-for-Reolysin/#:~:text=Monday%2C%20May%208%2C%202017%20FDA%20Oncolytics%20Biotech-%20announced,agent%2C%20for%20the%20treatment%20of%20metastatic%20breast%20cancer

[52] van den Bulk J, Verdegaal EM, de Miranda NF. Cancer immunotherapy: Broadening the scope of targetable tumours. Open Biology. 2018;**8**(6):1-10

[53] Biswas SK. Metabolic reprogramming of immune cells in cancer progression. Immunity. 2015;**43**(3):435-449

[54] Sampson JH et al. Tumor-specific immunotherapy targeting the EGFRvIII mutation in patients with malignant glioma. Seminars in Immunology. 2008;**20**(5):267-275

[55] Buchbinder EI, Desai A. CTLA-4 and PD-1 pathways: Similarities, differences, and implications of their inhibition. American Journal of Clinical Oncology. 2016;**39**(1):98-106

[56] Wang X et al. PD-L1 expression in human cancers and its association with clinical outcomes. Oncotargets and Therapy. 2016;**9**:5023-5039

[57] Zamarron BF, Chen W. Dual roles of immune cells and their factors in cancer development and progression. International Journal of Biological Sciences. 2011;**7**(5):651-658

[58] Landskron G et al. Chronic inflammation and cytokines in the tumor microenvironment. Journal of Immunology Research. 2014;**2014**:149185

[59] Dranoff G. Cytokines in cancer pathogenesis and cancer therapy. Nature Reviews Cancer. 2004;**4**(1):11-22

[60] van den Pol AN, Davis JN. Highly attenuated recombinant vesicular stomatitis virus VSV-12'GFP displays immunogenic and oncolytic activity. Journal of Virology. 2013;**87**(2):1019-1034

[61] Liu BL et al. ICP34.5 deleted herpes simplex virus with enhanced oncolytic, immune stimulating, and anti-tumour properties. Gene Therapy. 2003;**10**(4):292-303

[62] Tuve S et al. A new group B adenovirus receptor is expressed at high levels on human stem and tumor cells. Journal of Virology. 2006;**80**(24):12109-12120

[63] Uchida H et al. Effective treatment of an orthotopic xenograft model of human glioblastoma using an EGFR-retargeted oncolytic herpes simplex virus. Molecular Therapy. 2013;**21**(3):561-569

[64] Schenk E et al. Preclinical safety assessment of Ad[I/PPT-E1A], a novel oncolytic adenovirus for prostate cancer. Human Gene Therapy. Clinical Development. 2014;**25**(1):7-15

[65] Howard F, Iscaro A, Muthana M. Oncolytic viral particle delivery. In: Delivery Strategies and Engineering Technologies in Cancer Immunotherapy. Vol. 2. Massachussetts, USA: Academic Press; 2022. pp. 211-230

[66] Brahmer JR et al. Safety and activity of anti-PD-L1 antibody in patients with advanced cancer. The New England Journal of Medicine. 2012;**366**(26):2455-2465

[67] Bayat Mokhtari R et al. Combination therapy in combating cancer. Oncotarget. 2017;**8**(23):38022-38043

[68] Chaturvedi VK et al. Cancer nanotechnology: A new revolution for cancer diagnosis and therapy. Current Drug Metabolism. 2019;**20**(6):416-429

[69] Iscaro A, Howard NF, Muthana M. Nanoparticles: Properties and applications in cancer immunotherapy. Current Pharmaceutical Design. 2019;**25**(17):1962-1979

[70] Grimaldi AM et al. Nanoparticle-based strategies for cancer immunotherapy and immunodiagnostics. Nanomedicine (London, England). 2017;**12**(19):2349-2365

[71] Toy R, Roy K. Engineering nanoparticles to overcome barriers to immunotherapy. Bioengineering & Translational Medicine. 2016;**1**(1):47-62

[72] Bhat M et al. Nano-enabled topical delivery of anti-psoriatic small molecules. Journal of Drug Delivery Science and Technology. 2021;**62**:102328

[73] Bulbake U et al. Liposomal formulations in clinical use: An updated review. Pharmaceutics. 2017;**9**(2):1-33

[74] Bozzuto G, Molinari A. Liposomes as nanomedical devices. International Journal of Nanomedicine. 2015;**10**:975-999

[75] Alavi M, Hamidi M. Passive and active targeting in cancer therapy by liposomes and lipid nanoparticles. Drug Metabolism and Personalized Therapy. 2019;**34**(1):1-8

[76] Schlich M et al. Cytosolic delivery of nucleic acids: The case of ionizable lipid nanoparticles. Bioengineering & Translational Medicine. 2021;**6**(2):e10213

[77] Shah S et al. Liposomes: Advancements and innovation in the manufacturing process. Advanced Drug Delivery Reviews. 2020;**154-155**:102-122

[78] Barenholz Y. Doxil(R)—The first FDA-approved nano-drug: lessons learned. Journal of Controlled Release. 2012;**160**(2):117-134

[79] Russo D et al. Liposomal daunorubicin (DaunoXome) for treatment of poor-risk acute leukemia. Annals of Hematology. 2002;**81**(8):462-466

[80] Batist G et al. Myocet (liposome-encapsulated doxorubicin citrate): A new approach in breast cancer therapy. Expert Opinion on Pharmacotherapy. 2002;**3**(12):1739-1751

[81] Rueda Dominguez A et al. Liposomal cytarabine (DepoCyte) for the treatment of neoplastic meningitis. Clinical & Translational Oncology. 2005;**7**(6):232-238

[82] Silverman JA, Deitcher SR. Marqibo(R) (vincristine sulfate liposome injection) improves the pharmacokinetics and pharmacodynamics of vincristine.

Cancer Chemotherapy and Pharmacology. 2013;**71**(3):555-564

[83] Passero FC Jr et al. The safety and efficacy of Onivyde (irinotecan liposome injection) for the treatment of metastatic pancreatic cancer following gemcitabine-based therapy. Expert Review of Anticancer Therapy. 2016;**16**(7):697-703

[84] Pucci C, Martinelli C, Ciofani G. What does the future hold for chemotherapy with the use of lipid-based nanocarriers? Future Oncology. 2020;**16**(5):81-84

[85] Chen D, Zhao J, Cong W. Chinese herbal medicines facilitate the control of chemotherapy-induced side effects in colorectal cancer: Progress and perspective. Frontiers in Pharmacology. 2018;**9**:1442

[86] Ghajar CM. Metastasis prevention by targeting the dormant niche. Nature Reviews Cancer. 2015;**15**(4):238-247

[87] Rivankar S. An overview of doxorubicin formulations in cancer therapy. Journal of Cancer Research and Therapeutics. 2014;**10**(4):853-858

[88] Fassas A, Anagnostopoulos A. The use of liposomal daunorubicin (DaunoXome) in acute myeloid leukemia. Leukemia & Lymphoma. 2005;**46**(6):795-802

[89] Galmarini CM, Mackey JR, Dumontet C. Nucleoside analogues and nucleobases in cancer treatment. The Lancet Oncology. 2002;**3**(7):415-424

[90] Salehi B et al. Liposomal Cytarabine as cancer therapy: From chemistry to medicine. Biomolecules. 2019;**9**(12):1-19

[91] Zhang H. Onivyde for the therapy of multiple solid tumors. Oncotargets and Therapy. 2016;**9**:3001-3007

[92] Drummond DC et al. Development of a highly active nanoliposomal irinotecan using a novel intraliposomal stabilization strategy. Cancer Research. 2006;**66**(6):3271-3277

[93] Kang MH et al. Activity of MM-398, nanoliposomal irinotecan (nal-IRI), in Ewing's family tumor xenografts is associated with high exposure of tumor to drug and high SLFN11 expression. Clinical Cancer Research. 2015;**21**(5):1139-1150

[94] Zhang F et al. Nanoparticles that reshape the tumor milieu create a therapeutic window for effective T-cell therapy in solid malignancies. Cancer Research. 2018;**78**(13):3718-3730

[95] Du Y et al. Liposomal nanohybrid cerasomes targeted to PD-L1 enable dual-modality imaging and improve antitumor treatments. Cancer Letters. 2018;**414**:230-238

[96] Yu Q et al. Mild hyperthermia promotes immune checkpoint blockade-based immunotherapy against metastatic pancreatic cancer using size-adjustable nanoparticles. Acta Biomaterialia. 2021;**133**:244-256

[97] Nikpoor AR et al. Nanoliposome-mediated targeting of antibodies to tumors: IVIG antibodies as a model. International Journal of Pharmaceutics. 2015;**495**(1):162-170

[98] Li Y et al. EGFR-targeted liposomal nanohybrid cerasomes: Theranostic function and immune checkpoint inhibition in a mouse model of colorectal cancer. Nanoscale. 2018;**10**(35):16738-16749

[99] Lee H et al. (64)Cu-MM-302 positron emission tomography quantifies variability of enhanced permeability and retention of nanoparticles in relation to treatment response in patients with

metastatic breast cancer. Clinical Cancer Research. 2017;**23**(15):4190-4202

[100] Sun M et al. Boarding oncolytic viruses onto tumor-homing bacterium-vessels for augmented cancer immunotherapy. Nano Letters. 2022;**22**(12):5055-5064

[101] Iscaro A et al. Targeting circulating monocytes with CCL2-loaded liposomes armed with an oncolytic adenovirus. Nanomedicine. 2022;**40**:102506

[102] Yu J et al. Mannose-modified liposome designed for epitope peptide drug delivery in cancer immunotherapy. International Immunopharmacology. 2021;**101**(Pt A):108148

[103] Mohammadian Haftcheshmeh S et al. Immunoliposomes bearing lymphocyte activation gene 3 fusion protein and P5 peptide: A novel vaccine for breast cancer. Biotechnology Progress. 2021;**37**(2):e3095

[104] Varypataki EM et al. Efficient eradication of established tumors in mice with cationic liposome-based synthetic long-peptide vaccines. Cancer Immunology Research. 2017;**5**(3):222-233

[105] Su Q et al. Co-delivery of anionic epitope/CpG vaccine and IDO inhibitor by self-assembled cationic liposomes for combination melanoma immunotherapy. Journal of Materials Chemistry B. 2021;**9**(18):3892-3899

[106] Gu Z et al. Nanotechnology-mediated immunochemotherapy combined with docetaxel and PD-L1 antibody increase therapeutic effects and decrease systemic toxicity. Journal of Controlled Release. 2018;**286**:369-380

[107] Li C, Han X. Melanoma cancer immunotherapy using PD-L1 siRNA and Imatinib promotes cancer-immunity cycle. Pharmaceutical Research. 2020;**37**(6):109

[108] Ou W et al. Regulatory T cells tailored with pH-responsive liposomes shape an Immuno-antitumor milieu against tumors. ACS Applied Materials & Interfaces. 2019;**11**(40):36333-36346

[109] Kateh Shamshiri M, Jaafari MR, Badiee A. Preparation of liposomes containing IFN-gamma and their potentials in cancer immunotherapy: In vitro and in vivo studies in a colon cancer mouse model. Life Sciences. 2021;**264**:118605

[110] Kabilova TO et al. Antitumor and Antimetastatic effect of small Immunostimulatory RNA against B16 melanoma in mice. PLoS One. 2016;**11**(3):e0150751

[111] Liang X et al. A folate receptor-targeted lipoplex delivering interleukin-15 gene for colon cancer immunotherapy. Oncotarget. 2016;**7**(32):52207-52217

[112] Shelly S et al. Immune checkpoint inhibitor-associated myopathy: A clinicoseropathologically distinct myopathy. Brain Communications. 2020;**2**(2):fcaa181

[113] Huang YT et al. Immune checkpoint inhibitor-induced myasthenia gravis. Frontiers in Neurology. 2020;**11**:634

[114] Kalisz KR et al. Immune checkpoint inhibitor therapy-related pneumonitis: Patterns and management. Radiographics. 2019;**39**(7):1923-1937

[115] Tu K et al. Combination of Chidamide-mediated epigenetic modulation with immunotherapy: Boosting tumor immunogenicity and response to PD-1/PD-L1 blockade. ACS Applied Materials & Interfaces. 2021;**13**(33):39003-39017

[116] Hu M et al. Immunogenic hybrid Nanovesicles of liposomes and tumor-derived Nanovesicles for cancer Immunochemotherapy. ACS Nano. 2021;**15**(2):3123-3138

[117] Merino M et al. Dual activity of PD-L1 targeted doxorubicin immunoliposomes promoted an enhanced efficacy of the antitumor immune response in melanoma murine model. Journal of Nanobiotechnology. 2021;**19**(1):102

[118] Hei Y et al. Multifunctional Immunoliposomes combining catalase and PD-L1 antibodies overcome tumor hypoxia and enhance immunotherapeutic effects against melanoma. International Journal of Nanomedicine. 2020;**15**:1677-1691

[119] Elamir A et al. Ultrasound-triggered herceptin liposomes for breast cancer therapy. Scientific Reports. 2021;**11**(1):7545

[120] Kunte S, Abraham J, Montero AJ. Novel HER2-targeted therapies for HER2-positive metastatic breast cancer. Cancer. 2020;**126**(19):4278-4288

[121] Davoli A, Hocevar BA, Brown TL. Progression and treatment of HER2-positive breast cancer. Cancer Chemotherapy and Pharmacology. 2010;**65**(4):611-623

[122] van Broekhoven CL et al. Targeting dendritic cells with antigen-containing liposomes: A highly effective procedure for induction of antitumor immunity and for tumor immunotherapy. Cancer Research. 2004;**64**(12):4357-4365

[123] Saleh T, Shojaosadati SA. Multifunctional nanoparticles for cancer immunotherapy. Human Vaccines & Immunotherapeutics. 2016;**12**(7):1863-1875

[124] Carmeliet P. VEGF as a key mediator of angiogenesis in cancer. Oncology. 2005;**69**(Suppl 3):4-10

[125] Taurone S et al. VEGF in nuclear medicine: Clinical application in cancer and future perspectives (Review). International Journal of Oncology. 2016;**49**(2):437-447

[126] Kuesters GM, Campbell RB. Conjugation of bevacizumab to cationic liposomes enhances their tumor-targeting potential. Nanomedicine (London, England). 2010;**5**(2):181-192

[127] University, N. Irinotecan Liposome and Bevacizumab for the Treatment of Platinum Resistant, Recurrent, or Refractory Ovarian, Fallopian Tube, or Primary Peritoneal Cancer. 2022. Available from: https://www.clinicaltrials.gov/ct2/show/NCT04753216

[128] Chen J et al. Oncolytic adenovirus complexes coated with lipids and calcium phosphate for cancer gene therapy. ACS Nano. 2016;**10**(12):11548-11560

[129] Aoyama K et al. Liposome-encapsulated plasmid DNA of telomerase-specific oncolytic adenovirus with stealth effect on the immune system. Scientific Reports. 2017;7(1):14177

[130] Koshy ST et al. Liposomal delivery enhances immune activation by STING agonists for cancer immunotherapy. Advanced Biosystems. 2017;**1**(1-2):1-24

[131] Monpara J et al. Cationic cholesterol derivative efficiently delivers the genes: in silico and in vitro studies. Drug Delivery and Translational Research. 2019;**9**(1):106-122

[132] Yu MZ et al. Systemic delivery of siRNA by T7 peptide modified core-shell nanoparticles for targeted therapy of breast cancer. European Journal of Pharmaceutical Sciences. 2016;**92**:39-48

[133] Siefker-Radtke A et al. A phase l study of a tumor-targeted systemic

Nanodelivery system, SGT-94, in Genitourinary Cancers. Molecular Therapy. 2016;**24**(8):1484-1491

[134] Weng Y et al. RNAi therapeutic and its innovative biotechnological evolution. Biotechnology Advances. 2019;**37**(5):801-825

[135] Hou X et al. Lipid nanoparticles for mRNA delivery. Nature Reviews Materials. 2021;**6**(12):1078-1094

[136] Leung AKK, Tam YYC, Cullis PR. Lipid nanoparticles for short interfering RNA delivery. Advances in Genetics. 2014;**88**:71-110

[137] Aldosari BN, Alfagih IM, Almurshedi AS. Lipid nanoparticles as delivery systems for RNA-based vaccines. Pharmaceutics. 2021;**13**(2)

[138] Polack FP et al. Safety and efficacy of the BNT162b2 mRNA Covid-19 vaccine. The New England Journal of Medicine. 2020;**383**(27):2603-2615

[139] Guevara ML, Persano F, Persano S. Advances in lipid nanoparticles for mRNA-based cancer immunotherapy. Frontiers in Chemistry. 2020;**8**

[140] Billingsley MM et al. Ionizable lipid nanoparticle-mediated mRNA delivery for human CAR T cell engineering. Nano Letters. 2020;**20**(3):1578-1589

[141] Wang D et al. Acid-Activatable versatile Micelleplexes for PD-L1 blockade-enhanced cancer photodynamic immunotherapy. Nano Letters. 2016;**16**(9):5503-5513

[142] Zhao J et al. Polyester-based nanoparticles for nucleic acid delivery. Materials Science and Engineering: C. 2018;**92**:983-994

[143] O'Driscoll CM et al. Oral delivery of non-viral nucleic acid-based therapeutics—Do we have the guts for this? European Journal of Pharmaceutical Sciences. 2019;**133**:190-204

[144] Niu X et al. Bistable large-strain actuation of interpenetrating polymer networks. Advanced Materials. 2012;**24**(48):6513-6519

[145] Kowalski PS et al. Delivering the messenger: Advances in Technologies for Therapeutic mRNA delivery. Molecular Therapy. 2019;**27**(4):710-728

Chapter 6

Pulsatory Liposome: A Possible Biotechnological Device

Dumitru Popescu and Alin Gabriel Popescu

Abstract

A unilamellar liposome filled with an osmotic solution is introduced into a hypotonic aqueous environment. Because of the mechanical tension induced by the osmotic flow, the vesicle swells up to a critical size, when suddenly a transbilayer pore appears and the vesicle relaxing stage starts. A part of the intracellular material leaks out through this pore, and the liposome membrane relaxes and finally recovers. The swelling begins again and the liposome experiences a periodical process. For this reason, we have named it a pulsatory liposome. The swelling of the liposome is described by a differential equation. All the processes which contribute to the vesicle relaxing and its coming back to the initial size are described by three differential equations. The pulsatory liposome can be programmed to work a number of cycles, established before. The activity of a pulsatory liposome can be characterized by the following parameters: (a) number of cycles, the length time of each cycle, and liposome activity life; (b) the length time of the swelling stage and the relaxation stage for each cycle; (c) the amount of solute leaked out through the pore in each cycle. The pulsatory liposome may be regarded as a two-stroke engine.

Keywords: osmotic gradient, two-stroke engine, biotechnological device

1. Introduction

The transport of ions and molecules across cellular membranes is very important for many biological processes.

The pore appearance in lipid bilayers following some controlled processes may be an interesting way for transmembrane transport of molecules, especially large ones, with usefulness in some biotechnological applications [1].

There is a type of pore, called a stochastic pore, which can occur due to the structural and dynamic properties of the lipid bilayer [2–7]. On the other hand, the mechanical stretching induced in various ways in the lipid vesicle membrane may favor the appearance of transmembrane pores [8–13]. There are two interesting biotechnological applications that request the increase of membrane permeability: gene therapy and targeted special substances delivery. In the first application, the transport of DNA fragments through cellular and nuclear membranes is requested. In the second application, one uses special substances molecules encapsulated in vesicles, which must be transported to a previously established target location [14, 15].

In this chapter, we are writing about the dynamics of a pulsatory liposome. Such liposome makes a cyclic activity that may be described by a differential equation (the swelling stage) and a system of three-differential equations (the relaxing stage). This liposome may be programmed to work a certain number of cycles, settled in advance, and can release the drug molecules, in a well-controlled fashion. Also, we will calculate the amount of osmotic solute delivered during each cycle.

2. Phenomenological bases of a pulsatory liposome

Let us consider a unilamellar liposome filled with an aqueous solution of an osmotic solute. A solute for which the liposome membrane is impermeable is named osmotic solute.

This liposome is placed into a bath containing a hypotonic aqueous solution.

The osmotic flow of solvent determines three simultaneous processes: (1) the swelling of the liposome; (2) the dilution of the internal solution; (3) the stretching of liposomal membrane. The surface tension also increases at the same time as this liposomal expansion.

The swelling process is slow enough. The liposome increases up to a critical size when a transmembrane pore appears. This event is very important for liposome's life because it changes the sense of their evolution. The pore appearance is followed by two simultaneous processes: the pore dynamics and the outflow of internal solution from vesicle [16–19].

Figure 1 represents a cycle of the pulsatory liposome. In the first stage, the liposome swells from the initial state of radius R_0 to the critical state of radius Rc, when a transbilayer pore appears. In the second stage, the pore radius increases up to a maximum value, r_m, after that the pore radius decreases up to the pore disappearance. Simultaneously with the pore evolution, the liposome releases solution outside and relaxes until its radius becomes equal to R_0.

Both phenomena, the increase in pore size and the leakage of internal liquid, determine membrane relaxation due to a reduction in the mechanical tension of the membrane.

The internal liquid continues to leak outside the liposome, even after the edge tension equals the membrane tension. From the moment when the edge tension equals the membrane tension, the second part of the pore dynamics starts, and the pore radius reduces until the pore closes. Therefore, the liposome comes back to its initial size. In this new state, the liposome membrane is untensed but the solute concentration is less than in the preceding initial state. The dynamics of the liposome described above can restart over and over again. This cyclic process ceases when the osmotic gradient becomes equal to a critical value, which will be discussed below. In what follows we will describe a mathematical modeling of the two parts of a pulsatory liposome cycle: the liposome swelling and its relaxation.

3. The liposome swelling

Due to the influx of water, the liposome swells and its radius increases from an initial value of R_0 to a critical value of Rc. The liposome volume change is described by the following equation [20–22]:

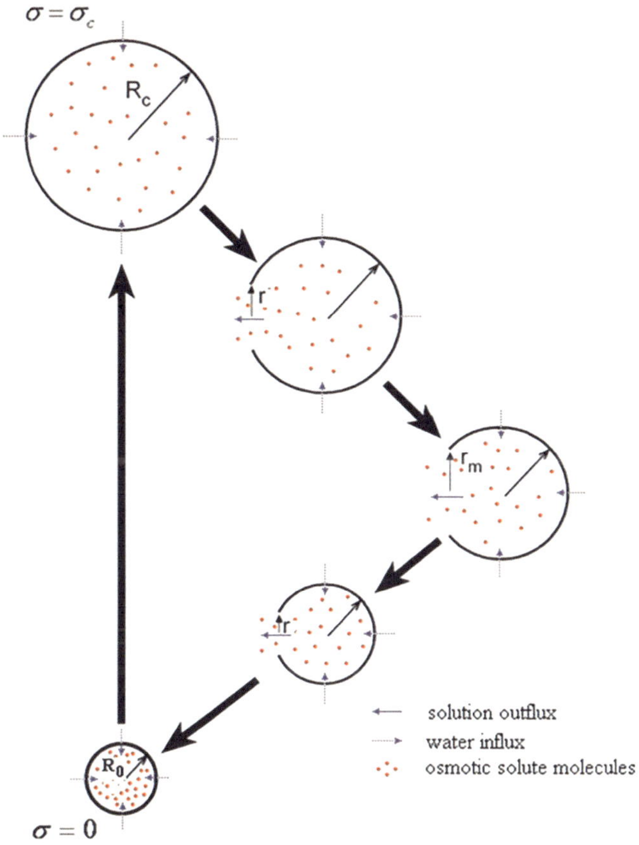

Figure 1.
A cycle of the pulsatory liposome.

$$\frac{dV}{dt} = \frac{P_w V_{\mu w} A}{\mathcal{R} T} (\Delta P_{osm} - \Delta P_L) \tag{1}$$

The notations from Eq. (1) have the following significances: V is the liposome volume, Pw (measured in m/s) is the water permeability through liposome membrane, Vμw is the water molar volume (in m^3/mol), A is the membrane surface area, $\mathcal{R}$ is the universal gas constant, and T is the absolute temperature.

The osmotic pressure, ΔP_{osm}, is equal to:

$$\Delta P_{osm} = \mathcal{R} T \Delta C_s \tag{2}$$

where ΔC_s (measured in mol/m^3) is the transmembrane solute concentration gradient.

The Laplace pressure is given by the formulae:

$$\Delta P_L = \sigma \left(\frac{1}{R - h} + \frac{1}{R + h} \right) \tag{3}$$

where σ is the tension of the stretched membrane, h is the hydrophobic core thickness, and R is the average radius of the liposome. Taking into account that the vesicle considered here is sufficiently large, we cut h, for now on.

According to Hooke law, if the radius of a spherical membrane increases from R_0 to R, the surface tension σ is:

$$\sigma(R) = E\left(\frac{R^2}{R_0^2} - 1\right) \tag{4}$$

where E is the elastic modulus for surface stretching.

During the swelling stage of the liposome, the solute amount does not change. Therefore, we can write:

$$C_{0s}V_0 = C_s V = C_{fs}V_c \tag{5}$$

where C_{0s} is the initial solute concentration; C_s is the solute concentration when the liposome has reached the volume V during the swelling process and C_{fs} is the solute concentration at the end of swelling stage, before pore nucleation when the liposome volume is Vc.

If one considers the external solute concentration is equal to zero, then $\Delta Cs = C_{0s}$.

With Laplace pressure formula and Eqs. (4) and (5) in mind we find from Eq. (1):

$$\frac{dR}{dt} = P_w V_{\mu w}\left(\frac{C_{0s}R_0^3}{R^3} - \frac{2\beta E}{R_0^2}\frac{R^2 - R_0^2}{R}\right) \tag{6}$$

In the above-written equation we have used the following notation:

$$\beta = \frac{1}{\mathcal{R}T} \tag{7}$$

By integrating the Eq. (6) one obtains the liposome radius R(t) as o function of time. The initial condition is: $R(0) = R_0$

The analytical solution to the Eq. (6) is:

$$(\alpha + 1)\ln\left|\frac{\alpha - 1}{2z - \alpha - 1}\right| + (\alpha - 1)\ln\left|\frac{\alpha + 1}{2z + \alpha - 1}\right| = \frac{8\alpha\beta E P_w V_{\mu w}}{R_0^2}t \tag{8}$$

where

$$z(t) = \frac{R^2(t)}{R_0^2} \tag{9}$$

$$\alpha = \sqrt{1 + \frac{2C_{0s}R_0}{\beta E}} \tag{10}$$

4. The liposome relaxation

The liposome swells up to when suddenly a transbilayer pore appears when the liposome reaches its critical size [23]. From this moment the liposome relaxation starts.

During this stage of the cycle, two simultaneous processes take place: the evolution of the pore from birth to its disappearance and the relaxation of the liposome from the critical state with the radius, R_c, to the initial state with the radius, R_0.

4.1 The differential equation for transbilayer pore dynamics

The change of the surface free energy due to the bilayer deformation following the pore appearance is dissipated into lipidic bilayer volume by the intermolecular friction forces characterized by the internal viscosity parameter η_m [24–26]. Equaling the two energy changes for the lipid bilayer, one obtains a differential equation for the dynamics of the pore radius [22, 27]:

$$2\pi r\eta_m 2h\frac{\partial r}{\partial t} = \pi r^2\sigma - 2\pi r\gamma \tag{11}$$

Pore opening is driven by the membrane tension, σ, and its closure by the line tension, γ.

According to the Hooke law, the membrane tension is equal to:

$$\sigma(R, r) = \frac{E}{4\pi R_0^2}\left[4\pi\left(R^2 - R_0^2\right) - \pi r^2\right] \tag{12}$$

The final form of Eq. (11) is:

$$2h\eta_m\frac{\partial r}{\partial t} = \frac{Er^2}{2}\left(\frac{R^2}{R_0^2} - 1 - \frac{r^2}{2R_0^2}\right) - \gamma \tag{13}$$

4.2 The differential equation of the internal liquid leak

After pore appearance, the internal liquid leaks out and the vesicle decreases its size.

The amount of expelled liquid in time unit is:

$$Q = \pi r^2 v \tag{14}$$

where r is the pore radius and v is the mean leak-out velocity of internal liquid.

The flow on time unit has to be equal to the decrease rate of the liposome volume, V_{lip}:

$$\frac{\partial V_{lip}}{\partial t} = Q - j_w \tag{15}$$

The outward flow velocity of the internal liquid one obtains by equaling the pushing out force, $F_p = \Delta P_L \pi r^2$, with the shear viscosity force involved in the outward flow, $F_v = \pi\eta_l rv$.

Taking into account, the formula of the Laplace pressure, the flow velocity is: $v = 2\sigma r/(3R\eta_l)$.

Here, η_l is the viscosity of aqueous solution.

The incoming water flow to the liposome through its membrane due to osmotic imbalance is:

$$j_w = P_w V_{\mu w} A(\Delta C_s - \beta \Delta P_L) \tag{16}$$

where $A = 4\pi R^2 - \pi r^2$ is the membrane surface area.

Taking into account the above equation, from Eq. (15) one obtains an equation for the vesicle radius:

$$4\pi R^2 \frac{\partial R}{\partial t} = \frac{2\pi\sigma r^3}{3R\eta_l} + P_w V_{\mu w}\left(4\pi R^2 - \pi r^2\right)(\Delta C_s - \beta \Delta P_L) \tag{17}$$

Given both Eq. (12) and the expression of Laplace pressure (12), the final form of the differential Eq. (17) is:

$$\frac{\partial R}{\partial t} = \frac{Er^3}{6\eta_l R^3}\left(\frac{R^2}{R_0^2} - \frac{r^2}{4R^2} - 1\right) + P_w V_{\mu w}\left(1 - \frac{r^2}{4R^2}\right)\left[C - \frac{2\beta E}{R}\left(\frac{R^2}{R_0^2} - \frac{r^2}{4R^2} - 1\right)\right] \tag{18}$$

4.3 The composition change of the internal liquid

The solute amount inside the liposome is modified by the solute efflux through the open pore according to the equation:

$$\frac{d(CV_{lip})}{dt} = -\pi r^2 Cv \tag{19}$$

which is equivalent with:

$$\frac{d[\ln(CV_{lip})]}{dt} = -\frac{Er^3}{2\eta_l R^4}\left(\frac{R^2}{R_0^2} - \frac{r^2}{4R^2} - 1\right) \tag{20}$$

The system of differential Eq. (13), (18), and (20) can be solved numerically using Euler's method to obtain the time dependence of R(t), r(t), and C(t) for the relaxing stage of a cycle. The time dependence of the liposome radius for the first stage of each cycle is obtained from Eq. (6). Also, the pore lifetime which is equal to the liposome relaxation time can be obtained.

5. The parameters characterizing a pulsatory liposome

The parameters that characterize the activity of the pulsating liposome are: (a) the length time of the swelling stage and the length time of the relaxation stage for each cycle, the length time of each cycle, and the lifetime of the liposome activity; (b) the quantity of solute leaked out through the pore in each cycle; (c) the number of cycles.

All these parameters can be obtained by solving Eq. (6) coupled with the system formed by differential Eqs. (13), (18), and (20) as a series of recurring systems of differential equations.

We have considered a unilamellar liposome inserted into a large box that contains water. In the initial state, the liposome radius is equal to R_0 = 19.7 μm [12]. R_0 is the initial value of the liposome radius for each cycle.

The liposome swells up to the critical state due to osmotic stress. When the vesicle reaches the critical size (R_c = 20.6 μm [12]), a pore suddenly opens. For the relaxing stage of each cycle R_c is the initial value of the liposome radius and σ_c is the initial value for membrane tension σ.

The value of the solute concentration at the beginning of a stage (swelling or relaxing) in the evolution of the liposome is equal to the concentration of the solute at the end of the previous stage (relaxing or swelling).

The initial concentrations of the internal aqueous solution of a non-permeating solute were C_{0s} = 11.5 mol/m^3.

The swelling time of the pulsatory liposome was calculated using the Eq. (8) in which $R(t) = R_c$. The membrane permeability coefficient for water p_w is equal to 3×10^{-5} m/s, and water molar volume is $V_{\mu w}$ = 18.04×10^{-6}m^3/mol. The two-dimensional stretch modulus of the lipid bilayer is E = 0.2 N/m [11]. Such unilamellar vesicles were used in experimental studies [11, 12].

The swelling time during the first cycle is τ_1 = 161.36 sec. The time dependence of the liposome radius is represented in **Figure 2**. The initial internal concentration solute of aqueous solution is equal to 11.4 mol/m^3.

The radius of the pulsatory liposome has a nearly linear dependence on time during swelling stage (**Figure 2**).

For the study of the relaxing stage of the first cycle of the pulsatory liposome working, we solved the system of three differential equations (13), (18), and (20) using Euler's method with a step size δt = 1 ms in order to see the time dependence of $r(t)$, $R(t)$, and C(t). Before numerical integration, all three equations were prepared by scaling the variables and parameters.

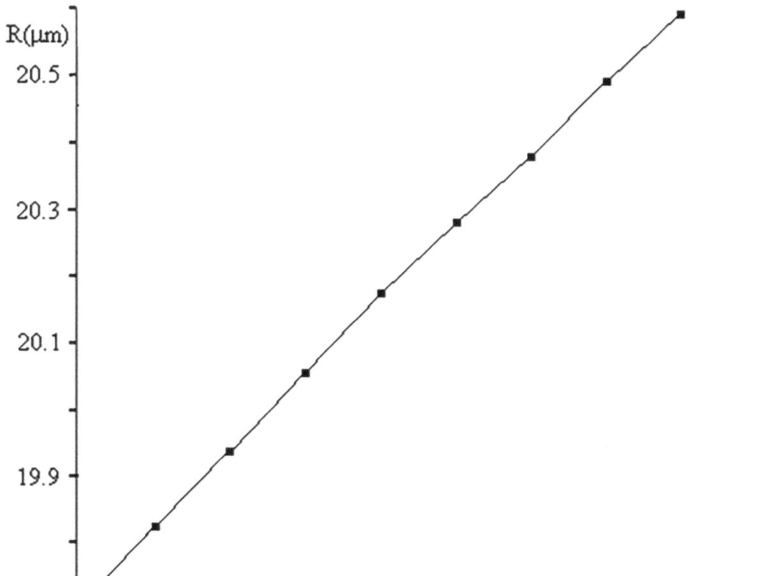

Figure 2.
The dependence of the liposome radius on time during the swelling process of a liposome inserted into water medium.

The initial conditions were: r(0) = 1.576 μm, R(0) = 20.6 μm, and C(0) = 10.04 mol/m^3 [23].

The liposome radius R(0) is equal to critical radius at the end of swelling stage. The initial solute concentration is equal to the solute concentration at the end of swelling stage ($C(0) = C_{0s}R_0^3/R_c^3$).

The edge tension was $\gamma = 8.1 \times 10^{-12}$ N [11]. The lipid bilayer viscosity was $\eta_b = 100$ N·s/m^2 [10]. The aqueous solution viscosity was $\eta_l = 3.2\times10^{-2}$ N·s/m^2 [10].

The pore evolution along its lifetime has drawn in **Figure 3**. In the first part of relaxing stage the pore radius increased up to r_m = 9.78 μm during t = 225 s, then its radius decreased until the pore disappeared in 1520 s.

The evolution of the pore size is plotted in **Figures 2–4**. We have drawn the pore evolution before reaching the maximum value of its radius (**Figure 2**), and after it reached its maximum size (**Figure 3**).

In **Figure 4** we have plotted the evolution of the vesicle size during the second stage of a cycle, that is during the relaxing of the vesicle.

For a more detailed image, we have drawn the vesicle radius evolution before and after reaching the maximum pore radius.

In **Figure 5** we have plotted the change in solute concentration during the pore lifetime when the aqueous solution leaks out of the vesicle. It is very interesting that the solute concentration decreases linearly during vesicle relaxation.

6. Programming the working of a pulsatory liposome

The internal solute concentration decreases along a cycle and with the cycle rank in sequence, and as a consequence, the osmotic pressure decreases too (**Figure 6**) [23, 28].

The liposome will swell up to its critical radius only if the osmotic pressure during the cycle is greater than excess Laplace pressure.

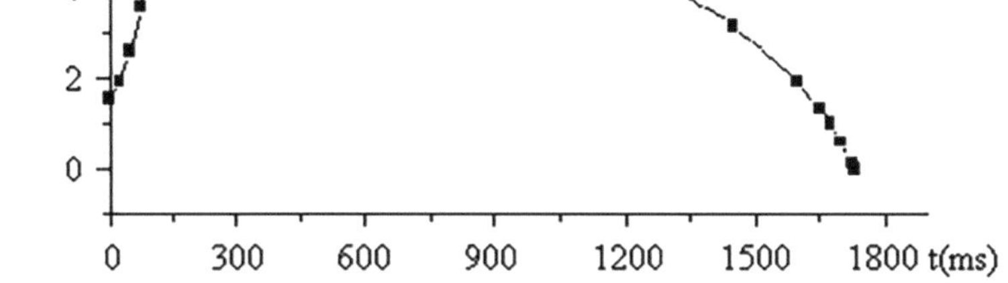

Figure 3.
The pore radius as a function of time for relaxing stage of a pulsatory liposome.

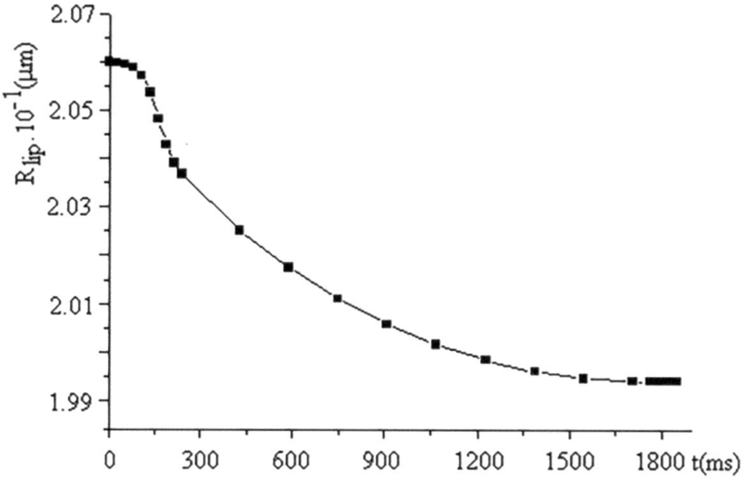

Figure 4.
The vesicle radius as a function of time during the relaxing stage of the liposome pulsatory.

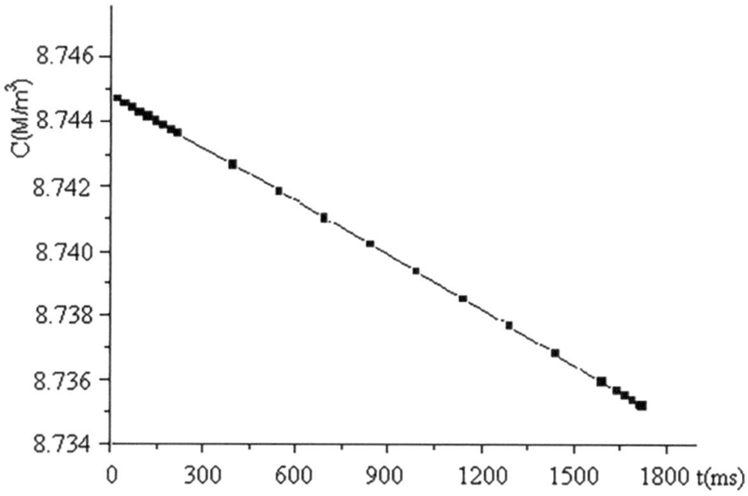

Figure 5.
The plot of the solute concentration inside of a liposome as a function of time, during the relaxing stage of the liposome.

$$\mathcal{R}T\Delta C_s \geq \sigma\left(\frac{1}{R-h}+\frac{1}{R+h}\right) \tag{21}$$

Given the condition (21) we can program a pulsatory liposome to work n cycles:

$$\mathcal{R}T\left(C_{sn}^{in}-C_{sn}^{out}\right)=\sigma\left(\frac{1}{R-h}+\frac{1}{R+h}\right) \tag{22}$$

where C_{sn}^{in} and C_{sn}^{out} are the solute concentrations at the end of swelling stage of the n-th cycle, inside and outside of liposome, respectively. Considering that at the beginning the solute external concentration is equal to zero, and the external medium

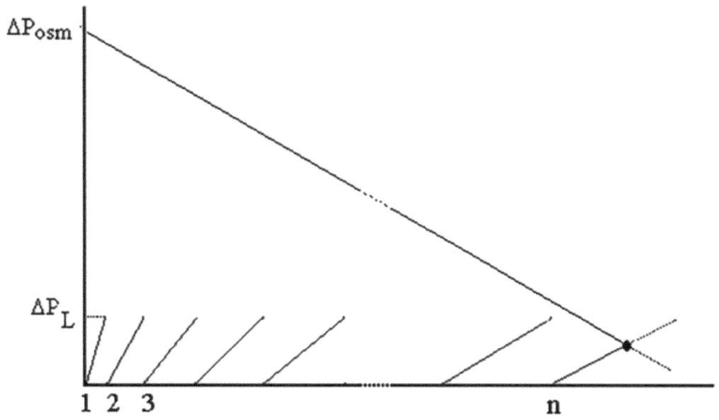

Figure 6.
The evolution of osmotic pressure and Laplace pressure during the working of the pulsatory liposome. The liposome stops working when the two pressures become equal (the black point on the figure).

composition is too less influenced by the vesicle running, we can take $C_{sn}^{out} = 0$. Taking into account that:

$$C_{sn}^{in} = f^n C_{so} \tag{23}$$

the condition (22) becomes:

$$\mathcal{R}Tf^n C_{so} = \frac{2\sigma R}{R^2 - h^2} = \frac{2ER}{R^2 - h^2}\left(\frac{R^2}{R_0^2} - 1\right) \tag{24}$$

where f is the reversal of swelling ratio ($f = V_0/V_c = R_0^3/R_c^3$), R is the radius of the sphere between the two monolayers of the liposome bilayer, σ is the monolayer surface tension, $2h$ is the hydrophobic core thickness, $\mathcal{R}$ is the universal gas constant, and T is the absolute temperature. Taking into account that the vesicle considered here is sufficiently large, we cut h, in order to obtain simpler formulae. R will be replaced by R_c and $\sigma = \sigma_c$. Therefore, it results from (24) that the initial solute concentration inside liposome, such as this liposome to produce n cycles, noted with c_{sOn} is equal to:

$$C_{sOn} = \frac{2\sigma_c}{\mathcal{R}TR_c f^n} = \frac{2E}{\mathcal{R}TR_c f^n}\left(\frac{R_c^2}{R_0^2} - 1\right) \tag{25}$$

The liposome studied in this chapter, filled with a solution with a concentration equal to 10.5 M/m^3 can work 20 cycles. If the internal solute concentration C_{sOn} of the solvate meets the condition $10.5\ M/m^3 \leq C_{sOn} < 12.14\ M/m^3$, then the pulsatory liposome will stop during the swelling of the twenty-first cycle.

The length time of a cycle is equal to the sum of swelling time and pore lifetime. The solute amount delivered through pore during a cycle may be calculated from the formulae:

$$q(n) = V_0\left(C_{sp} - C_{s(p+1)}\right) \tag{26}$$

where C_{sp} and $C_{s(p+1)}$ are the initial solute concentration before starting the p-th and (p+1)-th cycle.

7. Concluding remarks

The functioning of the pulsatory liposome is determined by the transmembrane concentration gradient of the osmotic solute and by the appearance of the pore through the liposome membrane. The transmembrane osmotic gradient is the motrice force, which causes swelling of the liposome. The pore changes the direction of the liposome evolution, bringing it back to its original geometric size.

Therefore, the pulsatory liposome can be seen as a two-stroke engine. The operating energy is ensured by the transmembrane concentration gradient of the solute. The solute is the fuel of the pulsatory liposome.

The number of cycles of the pulsatory liposome can be established according to the initial solute concentration. In other words, the pulsatory liposome is a programmable biodevice.

The solute (the fuel) may be a pharmacological substance or any other special substance.

The preparation of pulsatory liposomes with such properties and their delivery at a site of action remains a biotechnology challenge [29]. Some very interesting applications of pulsatory liposomes filled with drugs have been devised for targeting hepatic cells or the synaptic cleft. Endothelial pores (also known as fenestrae) control the exchange of fluids, solutes, and particles between the sinusoid blood capillaries and the space of Disse [23, 30].

Pulsatory liposomes, free or included inside other vesicles, may reach hepatocytes due to hydrodynamic effects of blood circulation [30].

The transient pores in liposomes could also be used for compensation of neurotransmitter deficiency in the synaptic cleft [31]. The pulsatory unilamellar liposome is an example of a bionic microengine, with potential applications in chemotherapy [32].

If the liposomal membrane is endowed with protein receptors of specific recognition, pulsatory liposomes can be used in chemotherapy as carriers and deliverers of drugs to certain sites in the body [32].

The range of systems and approaches that can be used to deliver therapeutics is advancing at an incredible rate. The advances in drug delivery have important implications for anyone working in healthcare. Therefore, we consider that, in the future, pulsatory liposomes may be used as special biotechnological devices for active substance controlled release [32, 33].

Author details

Dumitru Popescu[1*] and Alin Gabriel Popescu[2]

1 Department of Mathematical Modeling in Life Sciences, Gh. Mihoc—Caius Iacob Institute of Mathematical Statistics and Applied Mathematics of Romanian Academy, Bucharest, Romania

2 Faculty of Automatic Control and Computers, University Politehnica, Bucharest, Romania

*Address all correspondence to: dghpopescu@gmail.com

References

[1] Popescu D, Popescu AG. The working of a pulsatory liposome. Journal of Theoretical Biology. 2008;**254**: 515-519

[2] Popescu D, Rucareanu C, Victor G. A model for the appearance of statistical pores in membranes due to selfoscillations. Bioelectrochemistry and Bioenergetics. 1991;**25**:91-103

[3] Popescu D, Rucareanu C. Membrane selfoscillations model for th etransbilayer statistical pores and flip-flop diffusion. Molecular Crystals and Liquid Crystals. 1992;**25**:339-348

[4] Popescu D. Association probabilities between the single chain amphiphiles into a binary mixture in plan monolayers (II). Biochimica et Biophysica Acta. 1993;**1152**:35-43

[5] Popescu D, Movileanu L, Victor G, Turcu G. Stability and instability propertiesof aggregation of single chain amphiphiles into binary mixtures. Bulletin of Mathematical Biology. 1997; **59**:43-61

[6] Popescu D, Ion S, Popescu AI, Movileanu L. Elastic properties of bilayer lipidmembranes and pore formation. In: TiTien H, Ottova A, editors. Planar Lipid Bilayers (BLMs) and Their Applications. Amsterdam: Elsevier Science Publishers; 2003. pp. 173-204

[7] Movileanu L, Popescu D, Ion S, Popescu AI. Transbilayer pores induced by thickness fluctuations. Bulletin of Mathematical Biology. 2006;**68**:1231-1255

[8] Weaver JC, Chizmadzhev Y. Theory of electroporation: A review. Bioelectrochemistry and Bioenergetics. 1996;**41**:135-160

[9] Moroz JD, Nelson P. Dynamically stabilized pores in bilayer membranes. Biophysical Journal. 1997;**72**:2211-2216

[10] Sandre O, Moreaux L, Brochard-Wyart F. Dynamics of transient pores in stretched vesicles. Proceedings of the National Academy Science USA. 1999; **96**:10591-10596

[11] Karatekin E, Sandre O, Guitouni H, Borghi N, Puech PH, Brochard-Wyart F. Cascades of transient pores in giant vesicles: Line tension and transport. Biophysical Journal. 2003;**84**:1734-1749

[12] Brochard F, de Gennes PG, Sandre O. Transient pores in stretched vesicles: Role of leak-out. Physica A. 2000;**278**:32-51

[13] Trick JL, Song C, Wallace EJ, Sansom MS. Voltage gating of a biomimetic nanopore: Electrowetting of a hydrophobic barrier. ACS Nano. 2017;**11**: 1840-1847

[14] Verma IM, Somia M. Gene therapy—Promises, problems and prospects. Nature (London). 1997;**389**:239-242

[15] Zasadzinski JA. Novel approaches to lipid based drug delivery. Current Opinion in Solid State & Materials Science. 1997;**2**:345-349

[16] Chabanon M, Ho JCS, Liedberg B, Parikh AN, Rangamani P. Pulsatile lipid vesicles under osmotic stress. Biophysical Journal. 2017;**112**:1682-1691

[17] Levin Y, Idiart MA. Pore dynamics of osmotically stressed vesicles. Physica A. 2004;**331**:571-578

[18] Farago O, Santangelo CD. Pore formation in fluctuating membranes.

The Journal of Chemical Physics. 2005; **122**:1606-1612

[19] Alam Shibly SU, Ghatak C, Sayem Karal MA, Moniruzzaman M, Yamazaki M. Experimental estimation of membrane tension induced by osmotic pressure. Biophysical Journal. 2016;**111**: 2190-2201

[20] Popescu D. The Pulsatory Lipid Vesicle Dynamics under Osmotic Stress. Saarbruecken, Germany: Lambert Academic Publishing and AV Academikerverlag; 2012

[21] Popescu D, Popescu AG, Amuzescu B. Pulsatory liposomes—A possible biotechnological device for controlled drug delivery. I. The liposome swelling. Romanian Journal of Biophysics. 2010; **20**:37-46

[22] Peterlin P, Arrigler V, Haleva E, Diamant H. Law of corresponding states for osmotic swelling of vesicles. Soft Matter. 2012;**8**:2185-2193

[23] Popescu AG, Popescu D, Ion S, Amuzescu B. Pulsatory liposomes—A possible biotechnological device for controlled drug delivery. III. The liposome relaxation. Romanian Journal of Biophysics. 2010;**20**:223-234

[24] Alam Shibly SU, Ghatak C, Sayem Karal MA, Moniruzzaman M, Yamazaki M. Experimental estimation of membrane tension induced by osmotic pressure. Biophysical Journal. 2017;**112**:1290

[25] Srividya N, Muralidharan S, Okumu W, Tripp B. Determination of the line tension of giant vesicles from pore-closing dynamics. The Journal of Physical Chemistry. B. 2008;**112**:7147-7152

[26] Popescu AG, Popescu D, Amuzescu B, Maries E. Pulsatory liposomes—A possible biotechnological device for controlled drug delivery. II. The pore appearance. Romanian Journal of Biophysics. 2010;**20**:171-181

[27] Ryham R, Berezovik I, Cohen FS. Aqueous viscosity is the primary source of friction in lipidic pore dynamics. Biophysical Journal. 2011;**101**:2929-2938

[28] Imran A, Popescu D, Movileanu L. Cyclic activity of an osmotically stressed liposome in a finite hypotonic environment. Langmuir. 2020;**36**: 3659-3666

[29] Chabanon M, Rangamani P. Solubilization kinetics determines the pulsatory dynamics of lipid vesicles exposed to surfactant. Biochimica et Biophysica Acta. 1860;**2018**:2032-2041

[30] Popescu D, Movileanu L, Ion S, Flonta ML. Hydrodynamic effects on the solutes transport across endothelial pores and hepatocytes membranes. Physics in Medicine and Biology. 2000;**45**: N157-N165

[31] Popescu D, Zaharia CN, Ion S, Flonta ML. Compensation of the neurotransmitters deficiency in the synaptic cleft. Romanian Journal of Biophys. 2006;**16**:189-204

[32] Popescu A. Tratat de Bionica (A Compendium of Bionic). Bucharest, Romania: Bucharest University Publishing House; 2022

[33] Majd S, Yusko E, Billeh C, Macrae YN, Yang MX, J.; Mayer, M. Applications of biological pores in nanomedicine, sensing, and nanoelectronics. Current Opinion in Biotechnology. 2010;**21**:439-476

Chapter 7

Liposomes for Targeting RNA Interference-Based Therapy in Inflammatory Bowel Diseases

Iman M. Alfagih

Abstract

The discovery of RNA interference (RNAi) in mammalian cells in 2001 opened up a new class of candidate therapeutics for hard-to-cure diseases like inflammatory bowel diseases. The main challenge for the development of RNAi-based therapeutics is the efficient and safe delivery of RNAi since the RNAi machinery is housed in the cytoplasm. Among the various approaches to active targeting, liposome-based delivery systems are innovative and promising systems to transport and control RNAi molecules release and overcome some of their limitations. Many RNAis in lipid formulations have progressed through various stages of clinical trials, with the measurable improvements in patients and no side effects. For colon targeting, liposomes can be manipulated by different methods. This chapter discusses the progress in delivering RNAi molecules to the colon using liposomes.

Keywords: liposomes, targeted delivery, ligand, antibody, RNAi, mRNA, siRNA, inflammatory bowel diseases

1. Introduction

The discovery of RNA interference (RNAi) in mammalian cells in 2001 opened a new class of candidate therapeutics for hard-to-cure diseases like inflammatory bowel diseases (IBD). IBD refers to a group of immune-mediated chronic remission and relapse bowel diseases. IBD is classified into two subtypes: Crohn's disease and ulcerative colitis, with different etiologies and unknown causes. Crohn's disease causes ulcers and granuloma in the small and large intestines, as well as inflammation in the alimentary canal from the mouth to the anus. Ulcerative colitis causes an inflammatory response as well as subsequent ulcers and abscesses in the colonic mucosa. IBD patients are at a higher risk of developing colon cancer because of the emergence of chronic inflammation characterized by massive immune filtration and immune-mediated tissue destruction [1]. The prevalence of IBD has recently increased significantly. IBD has become the third most common disease in the world due to the development of chronic inflammation and a large number of immune cell filtration as well as immune cell-mediated organ destruction. IBD affects over 5,000,000 people worldwide. Currently, approximately 25 per million people yearly (developed countries) and 5 per one million people yearly (developing countries) are living with this

IntechOpen

chronic inflammatory and debilitating disease that necessitates lifelong treatment, resulting in a massive financial burden and healthcare system support [2].

Anti-inflammatory and immunosuppressive agents are the most commonly used therapeutic approaches. Nonsteroidal anti-inflammatory agents (such as mesalazine or olsalazine) are primarily used to treat mild attacks and to keep ulcerative colitis in remission. Unfortunately, the use of nonsteroidal anti-inflammatory drugs has been linked to a variety of side effects including nausea, diarrhea, cramping, headaches, fever, flatulence, rashes, and, in some cases, nephritis, pancreatitis, hair loss, and pancytopenia. In the treatment of moderate-to-severe IBD, steroidal anti-inflammatory drugs (such as prednisolone) are more effective. However, steroids' adverse drug reaction profile, which includes Cushing's syndrome, infection, adrenal suppression, sleep disorders, osteoporosis, and renal function impairment, limits their use in long-term therapy. Immunosuppressive drugs (such as azathioprine, 6-mercaptopurine, methotrexate, and calcineurin inhibitors) and the most important biological agents (such as infliximab, adalimumab, and certolizumab pegol) play an important role in the treatment of advanced disease stages. However, the use of immunotherapies is always constrained by a number of factors. For example, repeated administration of immunomodulators at high doses is always required, which may result in a series of autoimmune-mediated side effects, such as flu-like reactions and vascular leak syndrome, with significant individual variation [3, 4]. Clinical challenges include the drugs' limited efficacy, the high cost of antibody drugs, and the side effects or adverse reactions of corticosteroids and biological therapy [1, 5]. As a result, the development of new therapeutic strategies, such as the neutralization of proinflammatory cytokines, the use of anti-inflammatory cytokines, and the inhibition of neutrophil adhesion or T cell signaling, is critical [6, 7].

RNA interference (RNAi) is a common natural phenomenon that can be induced by exogenous RNA oligonucleotides (e.g., small interfering RNA or siRNA) and endogenous small RNA species such as microRNA (miRNA) and piwi-interacting RNAs. Since Fire and Mello's discovery of RNAi, new mechanisms of gene silencing and gene regulation have been elucidated, providing new tools for biological research and the development of new pharmacological strategies. Currently, the majority of RNAi research is focused on siRNA and miRNA. siRNAs are double-stranded RNA fragments of 21–25 nucleotides that can inhibit the expression of specific proteins by inducing the enzymatic cleavage of perfectly complementary target mRNAs. miRNA is a double-stranded endogenous noncoding molecule with 21–25 nucleotide segments and two nucleotide 3′ terminal overhangs. The RNAi technique modulates the expression of susceptibility genes as well as the secretion of proinflammatory cytokines associated with IBD, resulting in the therapeutic effects of mucosal restoration and immune balance recovery in disease sites. The RNAi pathway works by increasing the degradation of unwanted messenger RNA (mRNA) sequences and thus decreasing their translation. The main RNAi molecules being researched for IBD therapy are miRNA and siRNA. Both RNAi molecules interact with the RNA-induced silencing complex (RISC), resulting in the separation of RNA double strands by a RISC complex component (the endonuclease argonaute 2 protein, AGO2). The sense strand of RNA (passenger strand) degrades in the cytoplasm, whereas the antisense strand of RNA (guide strand) directs the RISC complex and binds to the target mRNA. In the case of siRNA, the antisense strand binds to fully complementary mRNA, resulting in mRNA cleavage. In the case of mRNA, the antisense strand binds to target mRNAs that are partially complementary to it, resulting in target gene silencing *via* translational repression, cleavage, and/or degradation (**Figure 1**) [8–10].

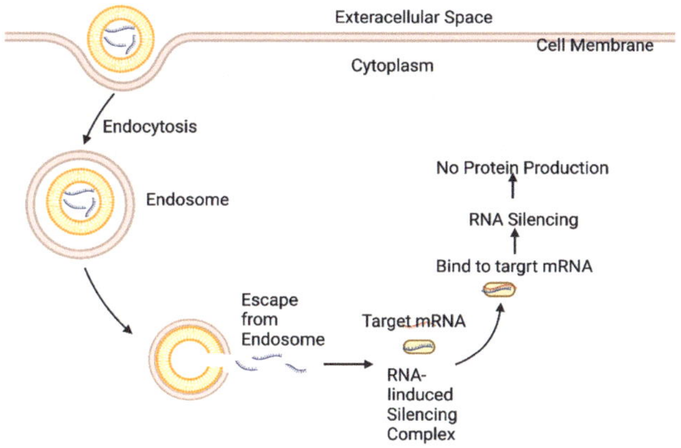

Figure 1.
Mechanism of RNAi molecule delivery via liposomal delivery system and RANi molecule gene silencing mechanism. Created with BioRender.com.

Formulation components	Target gene	Model	References
Lipofectamine 2000 (Invitrogen)	TNF-alpha	Murine	[17]
Lipidoids, cholesterol, DSPC, PEG2000-DMG	GAPDH	Caco-2 cells	[18]
Lipidoids, cholesterol, DSPC, PEG2000-DMG	GAPDH	Mice	[19]
DODAB, DSPG, HSPC, CF-PE	Model protein	Rats	[20]
DPPE, protamine, hyaluronan, antibody FIB504	Cyclin D1	Mice	[21]
HSPC, cholesterol, mPEG2000-PE, calcein, antibody (KN2/NRY or irrelevant human IgG), or haptoglobin	Cyclin D163	Mice	[22]
Ginger-derived lipids	IL-6, TNF-alpha, and IL-1β	Mice	[23]
Ginger-derived lipids	CD98	Mice	[24]

DSPC, distearoyl L-3-phosphatidylcholine; PEG2000-DMG, 1,2-dimyristoyl-rac-glycero-3-methoxypolyethylene glycol-2000; DODAB, dimethyl-dioctadecylammoniumbromide; DSPG, 1,2-dimyristoyl-sn-glycero-3-[phospho-rac-(1-glycerol)]; HSPC, Hydrogenated soybean phosphatidylcholine; CF-PE, cholesterol, 1,2-dioleoyl-sn-glycero-3-phosphoethanolamine-N-carboxyfluorescein; GAPDH, glyceraldehyde 3-phosphate dehydrogenase; DPPE, dipalmitoylphosphatidylethanolamine; mPEG2000-PE, 1,2-distearoyl-sn-glycero-3-phosphoethanolamine-N-[methoxy(polyethylene glycol)-2000] (ammonium salt); TNF-alpha, tumor necrosis factor-alpha; GAPDH, glyceraldehyde 3-phosphate dehydrogenase; IL-6, interleukin; IL-1β, interleukin-1β.

Table 1.
Lists of some liposomal formulations for colon-targeted RNAi delivery.

The use of RNAi in IBD models results in mucosal healing and the restoration of immune balance at the site of inflammation. RNAi techniques have high selectivity for intestinal tissues, a simple preparation method, and a low cost when compared with other IBD therapies [11, 12]. The main challenges for the development of RNAi-based therapeutics are efficient and safe delivery of RNAi molecules, endosomal escape, and entry into the cytoplasm. Moreover, RANis have a short half-life in the circulation, a

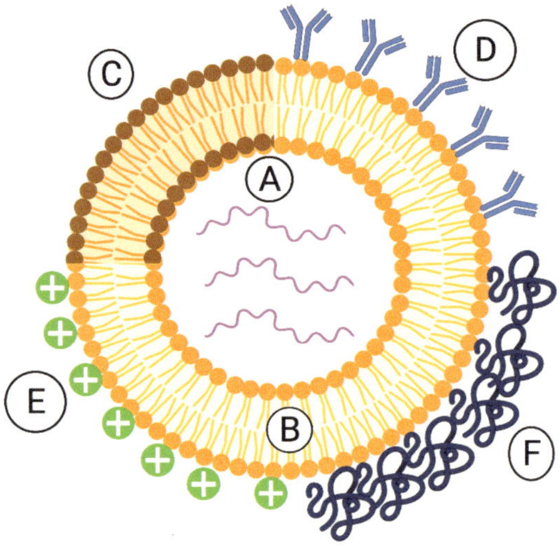

Figure 2.
Strategies for surface modification of liposomal formulations for colon-targeted RNAi delivery. A) RNAi molecules, B) lipid bilayers, C) natural lipids, D) ligand or antibody, E) coating with cationic polymers, F) coating with pH sensitive polymers. Created with Biorender.com.

relatively large size (13 kDa), an overall negative charge due to its phosphate backbone and degrade rapidly *in vivo*, necessitating targeted delivery to the site of action [13].

Among the various approaches to active targeting, liposomes-based delivery systems are innovative and promising systems to transport and control RNAi molecule release and overcome some of their limitations [11, 14, 15]. Many RNAis in lipid formulations have progressed through various stages of clinical trials, with the measurable improvements in patients and no side effects [16]. Alnylam Pharmaceuticals recently developed an FDA-approved first-of-its-kind intravenous dosage of siRNA-lipid nanoparticles, ONPATTRO® (patisiran), for the treatment of polyneuropathy [17]. Furthermore, 10 nanocarriers made with lipids are used in 12 ongoing clinical trials involving gene delivery, demonstrating the high potential of lipids nanocarriers for RNAi delivery [18]. Lipidic systems for RNAi molecules delivery have many advantages: The cell membrane is primarily composed of phospholipids (e.g., phosphatidylcholine) and cholesterol, making these natural lipids biocompatible. They have the ability to interact with the cell membrane and efficiently deliver the payload into the cell and can be purified or synthesized in large quantities [19]. For colon targeting, liposomes can be manipulated by different methods (**Table 1**, **Figure 2**). This chapter discusses the progress in delivering RNAi molecules to the colon using liposomes.

2. Targeting RNAi-encapsulated liposomes to the colon

2.1 Size and surface charge-dependent liposomes

The design of the liposomal surfaces in relation to the size, surface charge, and injury of the intestinal wall is the major challenge in the development of oral liposome-based carriers. As a result, a variety of modified liposome-based carriers are being tested in experimental colitis to determine the efficiency of accumulation and the improvement of clinical symptoms. There have been numerous studies that show the presence of macrophages and dendritic cells in IBD, and these can lead to liposome capture to a greater extent than tablets and solutions [20]. As a result, the size of liposomes is an important factor in drug delivery in IBD. Furthermore, electrostatic interactions allow nanocarriers of opposite charge to specifically target the charged surface of inflammatory tissues in IBD. Unlike the healthy regions, the mucosal composition of the inflamed colonic epithelium has a dysregulated mucous layer, a high degree of cationic proteins (transferrin, ferritin, bactericidal, or permeability-enhancing proteins (BMPs)), and accumulation of antimicrobial peptides (AMPs). This led to cationic charge build-up at the colitis surface. Thus, anionic nanocarriers as a delivery system can favorably adhere to the cationic-inflamed surfaces, release the drug locally, and prolong drug residency [21]. It has been demonstrated that positively charged liposomes better adhered to healthy mucosa, whereas negatively charged liposomes showed an increased adhesion to inflamed mucosa [3]. However, cationic liposomes have been the standard for siRNA transfection. These liposomes are used in commercially available transfection carriers such as lipofectamine. Lipofectamine was introduced in 1993 for DNA transfection and has since been optimized for siRNA transfection (oligofectamine, lipofectamine RNAiMAX). The phospholipid bilayer of the liposome allows it to cross the cell membrane and deliver its hydrophilic core of siRNA to the cytoplasm. When lipofectamine transfected, unmodified anti-TNF-siRNA prevented experimental colitis in mice following rectal administration [22]. However, cationic liposome delivery is complicated by toxicity concerns and requires efficacy improvement. Possible explanations include cationic liposomes made of cationic lipids, which are known to be membrane active. When incubated with cells, cationic lipids can disrupt the cell's or subcellular compartments' membrane function and integrity, resulting in toxicity. Another cause of toxicity could be the presence of the pH-sensitive lipid 1,2-dioleoyl-sn-glycero-3- phosphoethanolamine (DOPE) in the liposome. The intracellular fate of the complexes following uptake into the cells determines transfection success; the majority of the complexes are degraded in the lysosomes. DOPE may increase cationic lipid toxicity by destabilizing the lysosomal membrane due to the formation of an inverted hexagonal phase at acidic pH, which is typical of lysosomes. Furthermore, cationic lipids can become cytotoxic by interacting with important enzymes like protein kinase C. According to recent research, many cholesterol derivatives with tertiary or quaternary nitrogen headgroups can inhibit protein kinase C activity [23].

Many interesting types of liposomes with various physicochemical properties were prepared and tested in cell culture and experimental colitis models with varying degrees of success. An *ex vivo* study on neutral, positively charged, and negatively charged liposomes to target colitis induced by dinitrobenzene sulfonic acid (DNBS) revealed that anionic liposomes adhered to inflamed colonic mucosa twice as well as neutral or cationic liposomes. This adherence was dependent on the presence of 12,dimyristoyl-sn-glycerol-3-(phosphor-rac-(1-glycerol)) (DSPG, negatively charged) on the liposomes, whereas cationic and neutral liposomes did not significantly bind to the inflamed intestinal mucosa [24]. In a rat colitis model, negatively charged liposomes accumulated more in the inflammatory regions than cationic or neutral charged liposomes. These findings demonstrate that liposomes, whether positively or negatively charged, can interact with components in the GI tract, providing specificity in drug delivery. Unwanted electrostatic interactions, however, continue to be a problem in these systems. Charged liposomes have the potential to interact with oppositely charged GI tract components such as soluble mucins and bile acids [24, 25].

Despite the fact that anionic liposomes have been found to be specific in drug delivery, additional approaches are required to improve bioavailability in the colon.

Ball et al. prepared lipoid nanoparticles from amphiphilic lipid-like materials that form nanoparticles when complexed with cholesterol, distearoyl-sn-glycerol-3-phosphocholine (DSPC), and PEG-lipid. Three lipoids from a library of synthesized lipoids were chosen for their ability to target intestinal epithelial cells. The ability of one lipid nanoparticle, 306O13, to silence the housekeeping gene glyceraldehyde 3-phosphate dehydrogenase (GAPDH) in Caco-2 cells *in vitro* was then chosen [26]. Further studies show that 306O13 lipid nanoparticle were effective at gene silencing in HeLa cells *in vitro* across a pH range of 1–9, indicating that they may be stable across the pH range found in the GI tract. Pepsin and bile salts were found to reduce lipid nanoparticle GAPDH silencing in Caco-2 cells after they were subjected to simulated GI digestion conditions. Pancreatin and low pH (1–2) had little effect on silencing efficacy. Mucin at a concentration of 2% w/v in Caco-2 cell buffer was also found to significantly reduce silencing potential (90–40%). Lipid nanoparticles were found in mouse intestinal cells for 8 hours after delivery, and fluorescently labeled siRNA was found; however, gene silencing of GAPDH *in vivo* was not statistically significant. The low *in-vivo* efficacy could be attributed to uneven uptake. Working on uniform delivery across more epithelial cells may therefore yield better results [26, 27].

2.2 pH-dependent liposomes

Another approach for protecting liposomes from the harsh gastrointestinal environment is to coat liposomal surfaces with layers of polymers such as enteric polymers. Enteric coatings are well known for preventing liposome disintegration in the stomach, which improves absorption by allowing more liposomes to survive and be exposed in the small intestine [28, 29]. Liposomes are frequently coated with pH-dependent coating polymers such as methacrylic acid co-polymers (Eudragit®) for oral delivery. The liposomes coated with Eudragit® S100 exhibit appropriate pH response release characteristics when the polymer retains liposomal drug release at pH levels of 1.4 and 6.3 (resembling the stomach and small intestine, respectively), but releases the drug similar to plain liposomes NPs at pH 7.8 (ileocecal junction) [30]. Though pH-dependent liposomes have demonstrated excellent results in preclinical studies, the variability of pH in the colons of IBD patients suggests that a colonic drug delivery system based solely on gastrointestinal pH would be unreliable [31]. Despite the fact that pH-dependent liposomes have shown excellent results in preclinical studies, the variability of pH in IBD patients' colons suggests that a colonic drug delivery system based solely on gastrointestinal pH would be unreliable [1].

2.3 Active targeting-dependent liposomes

Polymers used to coat liposomal formulations have improved drug delivery to the colon after oral administration *via* pH-dependent release and mucoadhesive properties. These formulations, however, have a limited effect on the specificity of targeting to diseased versus healthy colon tissue. Surface modifications of liposomes with the coupling of ligands play a key role in drug delivery to more specific targeting to regions within the colon by exploiting disease-induced cellular changes in cell-surface receptors and proteins. Also, one of the more versatile ligands that can be affixed to liposome surfaces is the coupling of antibodies, particularly monoclonals, to create immuno-liposomes [32]. Veiga et al. used an ASSET (Anchored Secondary scFv Enabling Targeting) method, in which anti-Ly6c mAb is linked to liposomes, to target Ly6c + inflammatory leukocytes. The authors tested this strategy in a dextran sodium sulfate (DSS) colitis mouse model of inflammatory bowel disease using anti-Ly6c mAb coated or isotype control liposomes-formulated IL-10 mRNA, and they found that the liposomes-mRNA-targeted approach was more effective than the nontargeted approach [33].

Transferrin is a glycoprotein that transports ferric ions throughout the body. The transferrin receptor protein was found to be highly expressed in the basolateral and apical membranes of enterocytes in the colonic mucosa of IBD patients, as well as in the colonocytes of rats induced with colitis [34]. Transferrin receptor-mediated endocytosis is a normal physiological process that transports iron to cells. To create pendant-type PEG-liposomes, transferrin was coupled to the distal terminal of the PEG chains of PEG-liposomes. After that, transferrin -PEG-liposomes were injected intravenously into tumor-bearing mice. Transferrin-PEG-liposomes extravasate from the blood circulation and are followed by specific binding and internalization of transferrin -PEG-liposomes into tumor cells, leading to the delivery of their content into the cytoplasm *in vivo* [35]. Anti-transferrin receptor immune liposomes were found in higher concentrations in the mucosa of rats with dinitrobenzensulfonic acid (DNBS)-induced colitis than nonconjugated immunoliposomes in *ex vivo* binding studies [34].

An increased risk of colorectal cancer is the common feature of IBD. The chronic inflammation caused by these diseases can disrupt the cellular cycle, causing intestinal cells to replicate uncontrollably, potentially leading to tumor formation. Russo et al. used siRNA molecules to reduce the production of cellular cycle proteins CyD1 and E2F1 in explanted Crohn's disease intestinal tissue. Commercial siRNAs for CyD1 and E2F1 inhibition were encapsulated in Invivofectamine® leading to liposome nanocarriers designed specifically to silence CyD1 and E2F1 expression. As a result, the liposomes nanocarriers were able to reduce the amount of proteins associated with intestinal cancer in the tissue [36]. In a similar approach, protamine-condensed siRNA entrapped in a liposome modified with hyaluronan and coupled with a ß7 integrin-targeting antibody reversed experimentally induced colitis after systemic administration in mice. The condensation of siRNA with protamine allowed for a high drug load per nanoparticle (4000 siRNA molecules) as well as liposome protection against siRNA-induced interferon production. Furthermore, ß7 integrin-targeting antibodies coated on the outer surface of the liposomes provided selective cellular targeting, whereas cell surface integrins proved to be effective antibody targets for both nanocarrier delivery and uptake [37]. CD163 is a hemoglobin scavenger receptor that is overexpressed in the tissues of M2 resident macrophages as well as macrophages at sites of inflammation and tumor growth [38]. Etzerodt et al. studied CD163-binding monoclonal antibodies conjugated to the surface of PEG-liposomes to target CD163 cells and macrophages. PEG-liposomes mediated by antibodies significantly increased liposome uptake in both CD163-transfected cells and macrophages. Furthermore, the PEG-liposomal doxorubicin-targeted receptor CD163 exhibited strong cytotoxic effects on CD163-expressing human monocytes. The PEG-liposome mediated by CD163-binding monoclonal antibodies is a potential approach for targeting therapeutic agents to macrophages that support inflammatory and malignant progression [39].

2.4 Natural liposomes

There are two major drawbacks to synthetic liposomes. Before clinical application, each constituent of the synthesized liposomes must be tested for potential *in vivo* toxicity, and the production scale is limited. Liposomes derived from natural sources, on the other hand, are thought to be safe and cost-effective, and they may overcome the limitations of synthetic liposomes [10]. Extracellular vesicles have recently emerged as a more complex form of liposomes with a biological origin. Extracellular vesicles are nanoparticles encased in a complex lipid bilayer. They are released as exosomes and microvesicles from viable cells either on their own or in response to certain stimuli. Exosomes are formed within the endosomal system's multivesicular bodies. Exosomes are released when the multivesicular body fuses with the plasma membrane. Exosomes are reported to be between 30 and 150 nm in size. Microvesicles, on the other hand, have been reported to have sizes ranging from 100 to 1000 nm and are released directly from the plasma membrane [40, 41]. Using this approach, Zhang et al. isolated exosome-like nanoparticles from edible plants (ginger) using an eco-friendly protocol. The study demonstrated that ginger-derived nanoparticles increased survival and intestinal epithelial cell proliferation by upregulating anti-inflammatory cytokines and reducing proinflammatory cytokines (IL-6, TNF-α, and IL-1β) *in vivo* [42]. In another study, delivery of ginger-derived nanoparticles loaded with siRNA-CD98 was tested in colon-26 cells and successfully reduced the expression level of colonic CD98. Also, the oral administration of ginger-derived nanoparticles loaded with siRNA-CD98 reduced the expression of CD98 in the ileum and colon and thus may be useful for treating ulcerative colitis. Moreover, it was found that the effective dose of siRNA-CD98 delivered *via* oral administration of ginger-derived nanoparticles is approximately 10,000 lower than that of systemically administered naked siRNA-CD98 [23]. These studies suggest liposomes derived from natural compounds have immense potential in curing IBD.

3. Conclusion and future perspectives of liposomal formulations for colon-targeted RNAi delivery

The use of modified-liposome formulations as RNAi delivery systems has greatly improved RNAi molecule stability and therapeutic effectiveness. Because of their biocompatibility, biodegradability, low cost, stability, long-circulating times (PEGylated liposomes), and high encapsulation efficiency, nanoliposomes are preferred over other nanoparticle platforms as drug carriers. Furthermore, by attaching specific targeting ligands to their external surfaces, nanoliposomes can be functionalized. Several *in vivo* preclinical studies have highlighted the potential of modified-liposomes that retain RNAi activity at the target site. Despite the obvious advantages of modified-liposomes in terms of therapeutic development, target specificity, and reproducibility, their success from bench to bedside for RNAi therapeutics remains to be seen. Many RNAi in lipid formulations have progressed through various stages of clinical trials, with the measurable improvements in patients and no side effects. The development of modified-liposomes for RNAi molecules has enormous clinical potential as next-generation drugs.

Author details

Iman M. Alfagih
Department of Pharmaceutics, College of Pharmacy, King Saud University, Riyadh, Saudi Arabia

*Address all correspondence to: fagih@ksu.edu.sa

References

[1] Jacob EM, Borah A, Pillai SC, Kumar DS. Inflammatory bowel disease: The emergence of new trends in lifestyle and nanomedicine as the modern tool for pharmacotherapy. Nanomaterials. 2020;**10**(12):1-32. DOI: 10.3390/nano10122460

[2] M'Koma AE. Inflammatory bowel disease: An expanding global health problem. Therapeutic Advances in Gastrointestinal Endoscopy. 2013;**6**: 33-47. DOI: 10.4137/CGast.S12731

[3] Lautenschläger C, Schmidt C, Fischer D, Stallmach A. Drug delivery strategies in the therapy of inflammatory bowel disease. Advanced Drug Delivery Reviews. 2014;**71**:58-76. DOI: 10.1016/j.addr.2013.10.001

[4] Talaei F, Atyabi F, Azhdarzadeh M, Dinarvand R, Saadatzadeh A. Overcoming therapeutic obstacles in inflammatory bowel diseases: A comprehensive review on novel drug delivery strategies. European Journal of Pharmaceutical Sciences. 2013;**49**(4):712-722. DOI: 10.1016/j.ejps.2013.04.031

[5] Nielsen OH, Seidelin JB, Munck LK, Rogler G. Use of biological molecules in the treatment of inflammatory bowel disease. Journal of Internal Medicine. 2011;**270**:15-28. DOI: 10.1111/j.1365-2796.2011.02344.x

[6] Zhang J et al. Macrophage-based nanotherapeutic strategies in ulcerative colitis. Journal of Controlled Release. 2020;**320**(November):363-380. DOI: 10.1016/j.jconrel.2020.01.047

[7] Cabral H, Uchida S, Perche F, Pichon C. Nanomedicine-based approaches for mRNA delivery. Molecular Pharmaceutics. 2020;**17**:3654-3684. DOI: 10.1021/acs.molpharmaceut.0c00618

[8] Samaridou E, Heyes J, Lutwyche P. Lipid nanoparticles for nucleic delivery: Current perspectives. Advanced Drug Delivery Reviews. 2020;**154-155**:37-63. DOI: 10.1016/j.addr.2020.06.002

[9] Bobbin ML, Burnett JC, Rossi JJ. RNA interference approaches for treatment of HIV-1 infection. Genome Medicine. 2015;**7**(1):1-16. DOI: 10.1186/s13073-015-0174-y

[10] Chevalier R. siRNA targeting and treatment of gastrointestinal diseases. Clinical and Translational Science. 2019;**12**(6):573-585. DOI: 10.1111/cts.12668

[11] Campani V, Salzano G, Lusa S, de Rosa G. Lipid nanovectors to deliver RNA oligonucleotides in cancer. Nanomaterials. 2016;**6**(7):1-23. DOI: 10.3390/nano6070131

[12] Guo J, Jiang X, Gui S. RNA interference-based nanosystems for inflammatory bowel disease therapy. International Journal of Nanomedicine. 2016;**11**:5287-5310. DOI: 10.2147/IJN.S116902

[13] AlfagihIM, AldosariBN, AlQuadeibBT, Almurshedi AS, Tambuwala MM. An overview of nano delivery systems for targeting RNA interference-based therapy in ulcerative colitis. Current Pharmaceutical Design. 2021;**27**(25):2904-2914. DOI: 10.2174/1381612827666210617120302

[14] Tam YYC, Chen S, Cullis PR. Advances in lipid nanoparticles for siRNA delivery. Pharmaceutics.

2013;**5**(3):498-507. DOI: 10.3390/pharmaceutics5030498

[15] Zatsepin TS, Kotelevtsev YV, Koteliansky V. Lipid nanoparticles for targeted siRNA delivery - going from bench to bedside. International Journal of Nanomedicine. 2016;**11**:3077-3086. DOI: 10.2147/IJN.S106625

[16] Parashar D, Rajendran V, Shukla R, Sistla R. Lipid-based nanocarriers for delivery of small interfering RNA for therapeutic use. European Journal of Pharmaceutical Sciences. 2020;**142**(August):105159. DOI: 10.1016/j.ejps.2019.105159

[17] Hoy S. Patisiran: First global approval. Drugs. 2018;**78**:1625-1631

[18] Tyagi P, Santos JL. Macromolecule nanotherapeutics: Approaches and challenges. Drug Discovery Today. 2018;**23**(5):1053-1061. DOI: 10.1016/J.DRUDIS.2018.01.017

[19] Bruno K. Using drug-excipient interactions for siRNA delivery. Advanced Drug Delivery Reviews. 2011;**63**(13):1210-1226. DOI: 10.1016/j.addr.2011.09.003

[20] Ahsan F, Rivas IP, Khan MA, Torres Suárez AI. Targeting to macrophages: Role of physicochemical properties of particulate carriers - liposomes and microspheres - on the phagocytosis by macrophages. Journal of Controlled Release. 2002;**79**(1-3):29-40. DOI: 10.1016/S0168-3659(01)00549-1

[21] Chen F, Liu Q, Xiong Y, Xu L. Current strategies and potential prospects of nanomedicine-mediated therapy in inflammatory bowel disease. International Journal of Nanomedicine. 2021;**16**(June):4225-4237. DOI: 10.2147/IJN.S310952

[22] Zhang Y et al. Engineering mucosal RNA interference in vivo. Molecular Therapy. 2006;**14**(3):336-342. DOI: 10.1016/j.ymthe.2006.04.001

[23] Zhang M, Wang X, Han MK, Collins JF, Merlin D. Oral administration of ginger-derived nanolipids loaded with siRNA as a novel approach for efficient siRNA drug delivery to treat ulcerative colitis. Nanomedicine. 2017;**12**(16):1927-1943. DOI: 10.2217/nnm-2017-0196

[24] Jubeh TT, Barenholz Y, Rubinstein A. Differential adhesion of normal and inflamed rat colonic mucosa by charged liposomes. Pharmaceutical Research. 2004;**21**:447-453

[25] Beloqui A et al. Budesonide-loaded nanostructured lipid carriers reduce inflammation in murine DSS-induced colitis. International Journal of Pharmaceutics. 2013;**454**(2):775-783. DOI: 10.1016/j.ijpharm.2013.05.017

[26] Ball RL, Knapp CM, Whitehead KA. Lipidoid nanoparticles for siRNA delivery to the intestinal epithelium: In vitro investigations in a CACO-2 model. PLoS One. 2015;**10**(7):e0133154. DOI: 10.1371/JOURNAL.PONE.0133154

[27] Ball RL, Bajaj P, Whitehead KA. Oral delivery of siRNA lipid nanoparticles: Fate in the GI tract. Scientific Reports. 2018;**8**(2178):1-12. DOI: 10.1038/s41598-018-20632-6

[28] Gupta AS, Kshirsagar SJ, Bhalekar MR, Saldanha T. Design and development of liposomes for colon targeted drug delivery. Journal of Drug Targeting. 2013;**21**(2):146-160. DOI: 10.3109/1061186X.2012.734311

[29] Hosny KM, Ahmed OAA, Al-Abdali RT. Enteric-coated alendronate sodium nanoliposomes: A novel formula to overcome barriers for the treatment

of osteoporosis. Expert Opinion on Drug Delivery. 2013;**10**(6):741-746. DOI: 10.1517/17425247.2013.799136

[30] Barea MJ, Jenkins MJ, Gaber MH, Bridson RH. Evaluation of liposomes coated with a pH responsive polymer. International Journal of Pharmaceutics. 2010;**402**(1-2):89-94. DOI: 10.1016/J.IJPHARM.2010.09.028

[31] Ali Asghar LF, Chandran S. Multiparticulate formulation approach to colon specific drug delivery: Current perspectives - PubMed. Journal of Pharmacy & Pharmaceutical Sciences. 2006;**9**:327-338. Available from: https://pubmed.ncbi.nlm.nih.gov/17207416/. [Accessed: May 27, 2022]

[32] Hua S. Orally administered liposomal formulations for colon targeted drug delivery. Frontiers in Pharmacology. 2014;**5**(June):1-4. DOI: 10.3389/fphar.2014.00138

[33] Veiga N et al. Leukocyte-specific siRNA delivery revealing IRF8 as a potential anti-inflammatory target. Journal of Controlled Release. 2019;**313**:33-41. DOI: 10.1016/J.JCONREL.2019.10.001

[34] Harel E et al. Enhanced transferrin receptor expression by proinflammatory cytokines in enterocytes as a means for local delivery of drugs to inflamed gut mucosa. PLoS One. 2011;**6**(9):e24202. DOI: 10.1371/JOURNAL.PONE.0024202

[35] Ishida O et al. Liposomes bearing polyethyleneglycol-coupled transferrin with intracellular targeting property to the solid tumors in vivo. Pharmaceutical Research. 2001;**18**(7):1042-1048

[36] Russo I et al. siRNA delivery for control of cyclin D1 and E2F1 expression in Crohn's disease. Translational Medicine @ UniSa. 2017;**17**(5):25-33 Available from: http://www.ncbi.nlm.nih.gov/pubmed/30083520%0Ahttp://www.pubmedcentral.nih.gov/articlerender.fcgi?artid=PMC6067069

[37] Peer D, Park EJ, Morishita Y, Carman CV, Shimaoka M. Systemic leukocyte-directed siRNA delivery revealing cyclin D1 as an anti-inflammatory target. Science (80-.). 2008;**319**:627-630

[38] Baeten D et al. Macrophages expressing the scavenger receptor CD163: A link between immune alterations of the gut and synovial inflammation in spondyloarthropathy. The Journal of Pathology. 2002;**196**:343-350. DOI: 10.1002/path.1044

[39] Etzerodt A, Maniecki MB, Graversen JH, Moller HJ, Torchilin VP, Moestrup SK. Efficient intracellular drug-targeting of macrophages using stealth liposomes directed to the hemoglobin scavenger receptor CD163. Journal of Controlled Release. 2012;**160**(1):72-80. DOI: 10.1016/j.jconrel.2012.01.034

[40] van der Koog L, Gandek TB, Nagelkerke A. Liposomes and extracellular vesicles as drug delivery systems: A comparison of composition, pharmacokinetics, and functionalization. Advanced Healthcare Materials. 2022;**11**(5):2100639. DOI: 10.1002/adhm.202100639

[41] Doyle LM, Wang MZ. Overview of extracellular vesicles, their origin, composition, purpose, and methods for exosome isolation and analysis. Cell. 2019;**8**(7):727. DOI: 10.3390/cells8070727

[42] Zhang M et al. Edible ginger-derived nanoparticles: A novel therapeutic approach for the prevention and treatment of inflammatory bowel disease and colitis-associated cancer. Biomaterials. 2016;**101**:321-340. DOI: 10.1016/j.biomaterials.2016.06.018